Bulk Fill Resin Composites in Dentistry

Joseph Sabbagh • Robert McConnell
Editors

Bulk Fill Resin Composites in Dentistry

A Clinical Guide

Springer

Editors
Joseph Sabbagh
Department of Restorative Dentistry and Endodontics, Faculty of Dental Medicine
Lebanese University
Beirut, Lebanon

Robert McConnell
Restorative Dentistry
University Dental School and Hospital
University College Cork
Cork, Ireland

https://doi.org/10.1007/978-3-031-16388-3

This Springer imprint is published by the registered company Springer Nature Switzerland AG
The registered company address is: Gewerbestrasse 11, 6330 Cham, Switzerland

Contents

General Introduction

1

Joseph Sabbagh and Robert McConnell

1.1 Dental Resin Composites

Like all composite materials, dental resin composites are composed of several distinct elements including an organic matrix, an inorganic filler, and a silane coupling agent. They contain several other constituents include initiators, inhibitors, and pigments. Initially they were developed to replace silicate cements and unfilled methyl methacrylate resins for restoring anterior teeth.

Dental composites materials bond to tooth structure, are relatively stable, are very aesthetic with acceptable clinical performance in an oral environment making them well-suited for restoring teeth.

The early composites were two paste chemically cured products containing a BisGMA resin matrix with macrofilled fillers of quartz, borosilicate or glass particles of up to 100 μm in diameter [1].

Over the next three decades dental composites went through several modifications including changes to filler size; resin modifications; and curing methods resulting in materials with better handling properties making them suitable for restoring both anterior and posterior teeth.

Figure 1.1 Evolution of composites since the 1970s.

Despite these improvements polymerization shrinkage continued to be a major clinical challenge, especially when they were used in larger posterior restorations. This shrinkage is reduced when restoring anterior tooth as the outline of the cavities

J. Sabbagh
Department of Restorative and Aesthetic Dentistry and Endodontics, Faculty of Dental Medicine, Lebanese University, Beirut, Lebanon
e-mail: josephsabbagh@lu.edu.lb

R. McConnell (✉)
Restorative Dentistry, University Dental School and Hospital, University College Cork, Cork, Ireland
e-mail: r.mcconnell@ucc.ie

J. Sabbagh, R. McConnell (eds.), *Bulk Fill Resin Composites in Dentistry*,
https://doi.org/10.1007/978-3-031-16388-3_1

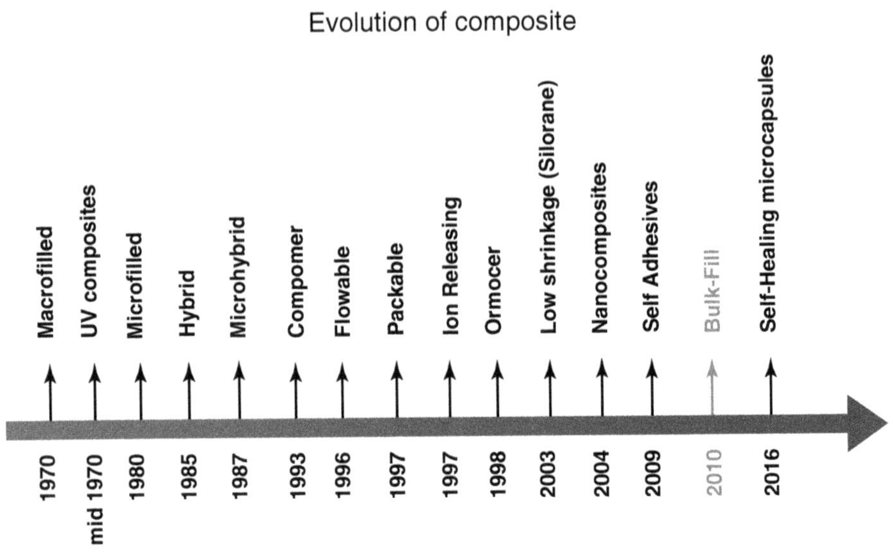

Fig. 1.1 Timeline of the development of major resin composites subgroups or categories

allows for better dissipation of the stresses along with incremental filling of the cavity. Furthermore, anterior cavities tend to be smaller than cavities in the posterior dentition.

Up to recently dental amalgam was the material of choice for posterior restorations.

Amalgam has been a very successful restorative material for decades notwithstanding the fact that it is unesthetic and inherently toxic. Using resin composite to restore posterior teeth is more complex than using amalgam.

With the endorsement of the Minamata Treaty in 2013 by several countries it became more urgent to address the reluctance by many clinicians to use resin composite posteriorly [2].

As more and more posterior teeth were restored or repaired with resin composites [3], research continued into the development of more suitable composite materials for posterior restorations. Various filler particles were added to improve the physical and mechanical properties of the material. These modifications did improve some properties of the material, however, polymerization shrinkage continued to be a major drawback, especially in cavities with multiple walls. Incremental placement of small quantities of the composite filling material posteriorly was recommended to dissipate the shrinkage. This technique was considered by some to be clinically difficult and to be more time consuming than when restoring with an amalgam material.

1.2 Cavity Design for Posterior Composite Restorations

Over the decades, dentists have used GV Black classification for cavities with the principle of extension for prevention concept. With the continuous evolution in dentistry and the introduction of new materials and techniques this classification of cavity preparations has been revisited several times.

A new cavity classification was published in 1998 in response to adhesive restorations by Mount and Hume [4]. This emphasized the principle of minimum extension. An FDI review of minimal intervention was published in 2000 [5]. Further publications in 2001 [6], 2002 [7], and 2003 [8] lead eventually in 2006 to a publication which introduced the SiSta classification of cavity design [9]. These publications emphasized that the main principle of restoring was to remove as little tooth material as possible. Only the caries part of the tooth required removal, leading to a minimal preparation.

Applying these principles when restoring posterior teeth with resin composite, the extent of the caries lesion will dictate the size of the cavity and not the physical properties of the material. No longer would the operator be required to cut a standard cavity design when restoring with a resin composite [10]. A minimal cavity preparation (Fig. 1.2) may leave unsupported enamel at the cavo-surface margin, at the proximal walls and on the cervical floor. This unsupported enamel need not be removed with a bur or chisel, making it easier to have a clean and non-bleeding surface to bond to, with no loss of healthy enamel (Fig. 1.3). Before restoring an interproximal cavity, the papilla can be protected by pre-wedging which will also assists in the development of a good interproximal contact [11].

The change to the modified cavity preparation is further supported today with a change in the disease process, the aesthetic demands of patients, and the heightened awareness by health care workers to retaining as much tooth structure as possible.

New clinical skills have been introduced into many undergraduate dental education programmes. Recent graduates are more experienced in placing resin composite in posterior teeth [12, 13].

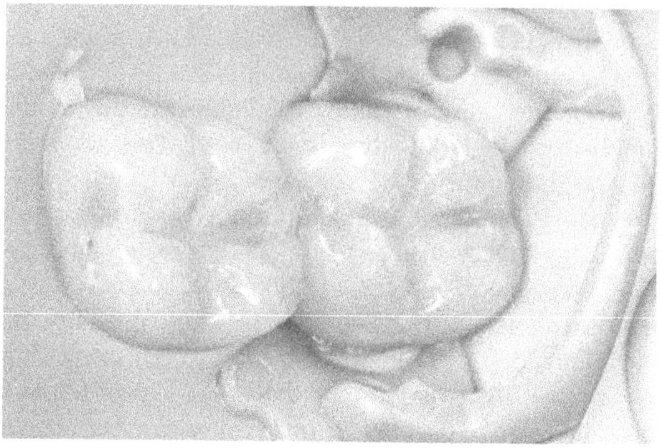

Fig. 1.2 Minimally invasive cavities

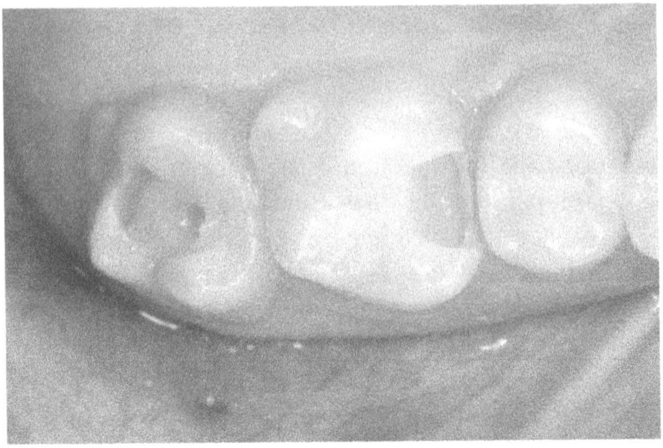

Fig. 1.3 Residual unsupported cervical enamel in the proximal box

1.3 Composite Placement

Liners/bases are not usually required for most posterior composite restorations as their use may prevent the bond of the adhesive resin to dentine. There is evidence that there is no difference in outcome in terms of postoperative sensitivity when a posterior resin composite is placed with or without a lining material [14]. Placement of a liner for therapeutic purposes should be used when required in areas close to the pulp. If a pulpal exposure occurs, evidence suggests that MTA is superior to calcium hydroxide [15]. Newer products such as Biodentine (Septodont) have potential use in this situation [16–18].

The Cochrane Library stated in a review in 2019 on the use of liners; *that there was inconsistent evidence regarding the difference between resin-based composite restorations placed with liners and those placed without liners when considering postoperative hypersensitivity. Further, there is no evidence of a difference between the use of liners or not regarding restoration failure. Despite the low quality of the evidence, we feel that this evidence is applicable when placing routine composite-based restorations in adult posterior teeth and that placing a liner is an unnecessary step* [19].

The clinician should be aware that stresses produced during polymerization can be a leading cause of adhesive failure, resulting in postoperative sensitivity, marginal staining, and recurrent caries [20]. This polymerization shrinkage can create stresses as high as 13 MPa between the resin composite material and tooth interface exceeding the tensile strength of the enamel often resulting in stress cracking and fracturing of the enamel [21]. When a resin composite is cured, the surrounding tooth structure may deform [22] and deflection can be significant depending on the filling technique used [23]. The higher the intensity of the light source, the greater the contraction force at the composite–tooth interface and so the use of high intensity plasma lights is not recommended. Lower intensities lights improve the marginal integrity of the restoration because it permits dissipation of the polymerization stress [24]. To achieve a clinically successful posterior resin composite restorations, it is vital to maintain the integrity of the bond and the marginal adaptation to tooth enamel and dentin.

The incremental technique is the preferred technique for restoring posterior teeth with composite resin and is recommended to dissipate the forces of shrinkage. The thickness is limited to 2 mm maximum for optimal polymerization and degree of conversion [25]. However, combined with a three-step total etch bonding technique, the restoration of a posterior cavity with resin composite using this technique can take much longer to complete than an equivalent procedure using dental amalgam [26].

Several benefits have already been outlined for using composite resin to restore posterior teeth. Composite materials in posterior teeth have the potential of extended survival of the restored tooth [26]. They support the use of minimum cavity design [27]. When the restoration is bonded to the enamel and dentine, they reinforce the remaining tooth structure requiring no additional retentive features or excessive tooth structure removal [28].

1.4 Bulk Fill Resin Composites

In 2010 a new class of material was introduced [29]. This was classified as bulk fill resin composite and intended to streamline the clinical placement of resin composites by allowing curing of 4–5 mm increments. These materials have enhanced light transmittance and depth of cure compared to conventional resin composites [30, 31]. They are a more translucent material with enhanced curing capability through filler modifications, incorporating high molecular weight monomers, and new alternative photoinitiators [32, 33].

Several currently available bulk fill materials have increased the filler size or have decreased filler content to minimize the scattering of light, thus encouraging light transmittance [34]. Adjustments have been made to the monomers and photoinitiators targeting improved optical properties, reduced polymerization shrinkage, and increased depth of cure [35].

Bulk fill materials are available in several formulations including flowable, full-body, and fibre-reinforced resin. Using self-adhesive bonding systems, the operator can shorten the bonding procedure and at the same time reduce postoperative sensitivity [36, 37]. When restoring posterior teeth with a bulk fill resin material, the total time taken to restore a posterior tooth is similar to that for a dental amalgam restoration [38].

Using bulk fill resin material to a primed tooth surface with less steps results in an enhanced bonded interface. Other clinical advantages include; less chance of contamination of the primed bonding surfaces with saliva or water droplets especially when most dentists do not use rubber dam isolation for placement of restorative materials [39]; in a time of airborne virus transmission, such as COVID-19 it is an advantage to the operator and other members of the health care team to minimize aerosol generation with the application of minimally invasive approach and prompt placement of the restorative material.

With bulk fill materials the resin matrix has been modified with fillers composed of non-agglomerated silica and zirconia particles. They have nanohybrid particles with up to a filler load of 77% by weight. Flowable materials generally have lower filler loading than the non-flowable products.

Fibre-reinforced composites are composite materials with three different components: the matrix (continuous phase), the fibres (dispersed phase), and the zone in between (interphase). FRC materials present high stiffness and strength per weight when compared with other structural materials along with adequate toughness [40].

Other modified bulk fill materials available to the practitioner include a sonically activated bulk fill material (Sonicfill, Kerr). Sonic energy contributes to increased fluidity with better distribution of inorganic particles which might be attributed to the amount and composition of the organic and inorganic matrix of this material [41].

Another modification to bulk fill materials include the use of thermo-viscous technology to heat the application gun which allows easier application of the material into the cavity followed by sculpturing of the resin (VisCalor, Voco).

Bulk fill restorative resins exhibit less polymerization shrinkage stress than conventional micro hybrid composites during and after light curing when used in Class II posterior restoration [42]. Teeth restored using conventional composite materials have significantly higher mean total cuspal movement values compared with teeth using bulk fill resin restorative material [43].

Cavity size and location may determine the choice of bulk fill material. Flowable materials may be suitable for narrow cavities or as a base for endodontic cavities. The lower viscosity materials allow adaptation to less accessible spaces due to plastic flow. Materials with higher filler load should be considered where resistance to wear and fracture are important [44].

It is difficult to compare different bulk fill materials currently available on the market. Research has identified a high variability in testing conditions, specimen dimensions, and curing protocols, combined with inadequate proprietary information concerning the materials' compositions. Instead of evaluating the individual properties of many materials, a comprehensive characterisation of a limited number of selected materials may be more beneficial for gaining insight into the relative strengths and weaknesses of the material [45].

Research does indicate that the use of high viscosity bulk fill results in a shorter clinical time when compared to conventional resins using incremental fill technique with no significant difference between the two groups in terms of postoperative sensitivity [46].

In a recent survey in the department of Restorative and Aesthetic Dentistry in the Lebanese University, the researchers compared the mean time taken by groups of operators with diverse clinical experience (fifth year students, specializing residents and clinical instructors in the restorative department) to restore posterior cavities. It was found that the bulk fill technique required the shortest time in comparison to the time required to perform the conventional layering technique.

The following chapters will update the reader on the current research and clinical techniques to achieve the highest quality posterior composite restorations. It will explore the differences between bulk fill and conventional composites and recommend the best adhesive regime to use with bulk fill resins. A major advantages of bulk fill materials is their depth of cure. It is crucial therefore that the operator understands what is happening within the composite resin when light is applied to the surface. Chapters will explore the various properties of bulk fill resin materials outlining their clinical challenges and recommend the best materials based on the literature/research and clinical experience of the authors. Finally, this book will address possible future developments for bulk fill resin restoratives exploring positive improvements for the clinician.

References

1. Aminoroaya A, Neisiany R, Khorasani SN, Panahia P, Das O, Madry H, Cucchiarinid M, Ramakrishnae S. A review of dental composites: challenges, chemistry aspects, filler influences, and future insights. Compos Part B. 2021;216:108852.
2. United Nations Environment Programme (UNEP). Global Mercury Assessment 2013: sources, emissions, releases and environmental transport. Geneva: UNEP Chemicals Branch; 2013.
3. Kopperud SE, Staxrud F, Espelid I, Bjørg Tveit A. The post-amalgam era: Norwegian dentists' experiences with composite resins and repair of defective amalgam restorations. Int J Environ Res Public Health. 2016;13(4):441.
4. Mount GJ, Hume WR. A new cavity classification. Aust Dent J. 1998;43:153–9.
5. Tyas MJ, Anusavice KJ, Frencken JE, Mount GJ. Minimal intervention dentistry–a review. FDI commission project 1–97. Int Dent J. 2000;50(1):1–12.
6. Lasfargues JJ, Kaleka R, Louis JJ. A new therapeutic classification of cavities. Quintessence Int. 2001;32(2):97.
7. Sathyanarayanan R, Caraunnanidy U. Classification and management of dental caries. New concepts. Indian J Dent Res. 2002;1(1):21–5.
8. Burke FJ. From extension for prevention to prevention of extension (minimal intervention dentistry). Dent Update. 2003;30(9):492–8.
9. Mount GJ, Tyas JM, Duke ES, Hume WR, Lasfargues JJ, Kaleka R. A proposal for a new classification of lesions of exposed tooth surfaces. Int Dent J. 2006;56(2):82–91.
10. Kidd E. Clinical threshold for caries removal. Dent Clin N Am. 2010;54:541–9.
11. Sabbagh J, McConnell RJ, McConnell MC. Posterior composites: update on cavities and filling techniques. J Dent. 2017;57:86–90.
12. Wilson NH, Lynch CD. The teaching of posterior resin composites: planning for the future based on 25 years of research. J Dent. 2014;42:503–16.
13. Lynch CD, Frazier KB, McConnell RJ, Blum IR, Wilson NHF. State-of-the-art techniques in operative dentistry: contemporary teaching of posterior composites in UK and Irish dental schools. Br Dent J. 2010;209:120–36.
14. Burrow MF, Banomyong D, Harnirattisai C, Messer HH. Effect of glassionomer cement lining on postoperative sensitivity in occlusal cavities restored with resin composite—a randomized clinical trial. Open Dent. 2009;34:648–55. [24] L. Bjørndal, C. Reit, G. Bruun, M. Markvart, M. Kjaeldgaard, P. Näsman, M.
15. Hilton TJ, Ferracane JL, Mancl L. Northwest practice-based research collaborative in evidence-based dentistry (NWP): comparison of CaOH with MTA for direct pulp capping: a PBRN randomized clinical trial. J Dent Res. 2013;92:16S–22S.
16. Mouawad S, Artine S, Hajjar P, McConnell R, Fahd J, Sabbagh J. Frequently asked questions in direct pulp capping. Dent Update. 2014;41(4):298–300. 302–4, 298–304.

17. Hashem D, Mannocci F, Patel S, Manoharan A, Brown JE, Watson TF, Banerjee A. Clinical and radiographic assessment of the efficacy of calcium silicate indirect pulp capping: a randomized controlled clinical trial. J Dent Res. 2015;94(4):562–8.
18. Tziafa C, Koliniotou-Koumpia E, Papadimitriou S, Tziafas D. Dentinogenic activity of biodentine in deep cavities of miniature swine teeth. J Endod. 2015;41(7):1161–6.
19. Schenkel AB, Veitz-Keenan A. Dental cavity liners for class I and class II resin-based composite restorations. Cochrane Database Syst Rev. 2019;3(3):CD010526. https://doi.org/10.1002/14651858.CD010526.pub3.
20. Condon JR, Ferracane JL. Assessing the effect of composite formulation on polymerization stress. J Am Dent Assoc. 2000;131(9):497–503.
21. Craig RG, Powers JM. Restorative dental materials. 11th ed. St Louis: Mosby; 2002. p. 239.
22. Tantbirojn D, Versluis A, Pintado MR, et al. Tooth deformation patterns in molars after composite restoration. Dent Mater. 2004;20:535–42.
23. Gonzalez-Lopez S, Lucena-Martin C, de Haro-Gasquet F, et al. Influence of different composite restoration techniques on cuspal deflection: an in vitro study. Oper Dent. 2004;29:656–60.
24. Alonso RC, Cunha LG, Correr GM, et al. Association of photoactivation methods and low modulus liners on marginal adaptation of composite restorations. Acta Odontol Scand. 2004;62:298–304.
25. Dietschi D, Argente A, Krejci I, Mandikos M. In vitro performance of class I and II composite restorations: a literature review on nondestructive laboratory trials–part I. Oper Dent. 2013;38(5):166–81.
26. Lynch CD, Opdam NJ, Hickel R, et al. Guidance on posterior resin composites: academy of operative dentistry–European section. J Dent. 2014;42:377–83.
27. Wilson NHF. Minimally invasive dentistry–the management of caries. London: Quintessence; 2007.
28. Lynch CD. Successful posterior resin composites. London: Quintessence; 2008.
29. Miletic V. Development of dental composites. In: Miletic V, editor. Dental composite materials for direct restorations. Cham: Springer; 2018. https://doi.org/10.1007/978-3-319-60961-4_1.
30. Bucuta S, Ilie N. Light transmittance, and micro-mechanical properties of bulk fill vs. conventional resin-based composites. Clin Oral Investig. 2014;18(8):1991–2000.
31. Zorzin J, Maier E, Harre S, Fey T, Belli R, Lohbauer U, et al. Bulk-fill resin composites: polymerization properties and extended light curing. Dent Mater. 2015;31(3):293–301.
32. Ersen KA, Gurbuz O, Ozcan M. Evaluation of polymerization shrinkage of bulk-fill resin composites using microcomputed tomography. Clin Oral Investig. 2020;24(5):1687–93.
33. Ilie N, Bucuta S, Draenert M. Bulk-fill resin-based composites: an *in vitro* assessment of their mechanical performance. Oper Dent. 2013;38(6):618–25.
34. Fronza BM, Ayres AP, Pacheco RR, Rueggeberg FA, Dias CT, Giannini M. Characterization of inorganic filler content, mechanical properties, and light transmission of bulk-fill resin composites. Oper Dent. 2017;42(4):445–55.
35. Ilie N, Stark K. Curing behaviour of high-viscosity bulk-fill composites. J Dent. 2014;42(8):977–85.
36. Alex G. Universal adhesives: the next evolution in adhesive dentistry? Compend Contin Educ Dent. 2015;36(1):15–26.
37. Perdigão J, Frankenberger R, Rosa BT, Breschi L. New trends in dentin/enamel adhesion. Am J Dent. 2000;13:25D–30D.
38. Do T, Church B, Veríssimo C, Hackmyer SP, Tantbirojn D, Simon JF, Versluis A. Cuspal flexure, depth-of-cure, and bond integrity of bulk-fill composites. Pediatr Dent. 2014;36(7):468–73.
39. Sabbagh J, McConnell RJ, Clancy McConnell M. Posterior composites: update on cavities and filling techniques. J Dent. 2017;57:86–90.
40. Scribante A, Vallittu PK, Özcan M. Fiber-reinforced composites for dental applications. Biomed Res Int. 2018;2018:4734986. 2 pages
41. Penha S, Souza A-F, dos Santos M-J, dos Santos-Almeida Júnior L-J, Tavarez R-R-DJ, Firoozmand L-M. Could sonic delivery of bulk-fill resins improve the bond strength and cure depth in extended size class I cavities? J Clin Exp Dent. 2020;12:e1131.

42. Lins RBE, Arisilde S, Osorio JH, Cordeiro CMB, Yanikian CRF, Bicalho AA, Stape THS, Soares CJ, Martins LRM. Biomechanical behavior of bulk-fill resin composites in class II restorations. J Mech Behav Biomed Mater. 2019;98:255–61.
43. Politi I, McHugh LEJ, Al-Fodeh RS, Fleming GJP. Modification of the restoration protocol for resin-based composite (RBC) restoratives (conventional and bulk fill) on cuspal movement and microleakage score in molar teeth. Dent Mater. 2018;34(9):1271–7.
44. Van Ende A, De Munck J, Lise DP, Van Meerbeek B. J Adhes Dent. 2017;2017(19):95–109.
45. Haugen HJ, Marovic D, Par M, Le Thieu MK, Reseland JE, Johnsen GF. Bulk fill composites have similar performance to conventional dental composites. Int J Mol Sci. 2020;21(14):5136.
46. Bellinaso MD, Soares FZM, Rocha RO. Do bulk-fill resins decrease the restorative time in posterior teeth? A systematic review and meta-analysis of in vitro studies. J Investig Clin Dent. 2019;10(4):e12463.

What Are Bulk Fill (BF) Composites and How Do They Differ from Non-BF Composites?

2

Joseph Sabbagh, Jean Claude Fahd, Layal El Masri, and Paul Nahas

2.1 What Are Bulk Fill Composites?

Since resin composites were introduced over 50 years ago they have been increasingly used for the restoration of anterior and posterior teeth [1]. Two factors have promoted this increase in use; the perceived risk of toxicity caused by amalgam restorations and the patient demand for aesthetic restorations [2]. Despite the improvements made to the materials, polymerization shrinkage remains their main shortcoming, affecting their long-term stability [3]. In general, resin composites have volumetric shrinkage values that range from less than 1% up to 6%, depending on their formulation and curing settings [4]. Various clinical approaches have been proposed to overcome this problem and to obtain an adequate degree of conversion, such as the use of "incremental layering technique." This method involves the application of resin composite in layers of 2 mm for anterior and posterior restorations [5]. The layering technique or stratification using different opacities is used for aesthetic purposes, and has been the state of the art for the last decade. Despite its aesthetic outcomes and reduction in polymerization shrinkage, it is time consuming. Completing a posterior composite restoration, can take up to 2.5 more time as compared to placing an amalgam, as it involves several steps including the application of the adhesive system [6]. As well as polymerization shrinkage the dentist can face other clinical difficulties including the establishment of an adequate contact point and occasionally post-operative sensitivity.

J. Sabbagh (✉) · J. C. Fahd · L. El Masri · P. Nahas
Restorative and Aesthetic Dentistry and Endodontic Department, Faculty of Dental Medicine, Lebanese University, Beirut, Lebanon
e-mail: josephsabbagh@ul.edu.lb; jeanfahd@ul.edu.lb; l.almasri@ul.edu.lb; paulnahas@ul.edu.lb

J. Sabbagh, R. McConnell (eds.), *Bulk Fill Resin Composites in Dentistry*,
https://doi.org/10.1007/978-3-031-16388-3_2

Today more than 200 brands of resin composites from different manufacturers are available on the market. In the last decade, many types of resin-based materials have been launched, but not all of them have been successful including Compomer, packable composites, siloranes, and self-adhesive composites. On the other hand, flowable composites, nanocomposites, and more recently, bulk fill resin composites have been shown to be clinically suitable.

Many bulk fill materials for posterior restorations are available from different manufacturers as given in Table 2.1. The different classifications of bulk fill materials will be detailed later in this chapter.

Table 2.1 List of available bulk fill resin composite from different manufacturers

	Composite BF	Manufacturer	Shades available
Bulk Fill RBC			
1	Filtek Bulk Fill	3M ESPE	A1, A2, A3, B1, C2
2	Filtek one bulk fill	3M ESPE	A1, A2, A3, B1, C2
3	Tetric Evo Ceram Bulk Fill	Ivoclar-Vivadent	IVA (Universal A shade) IVB (Universal B shade) IVW (white for light coloured or deciduous teeth)
4	Tetric N-Ceram Bulk Fill	Ivoclar-Vivadent	IVA, IVB, IVW
5	X-tra fil	VOCO	Universal shade
6	Aura Bulk Fill	SDI dental	BKF
7	Beautifil bulk restorative GIOMER	SHOFU	Universal, A
8	EverX Posterior	GC	Universal shade (transparent)
9	Dexta Fill Bulk	Dexter	A, U
10	Ecosite Bulk Fill	DMG	Light, universal, contrast for core build ups
11	Opus Bulk fill APS	FGM	A1, A2, A3
12	Reveal HD Bulk Fill	BISCO	A1, A2, A3, B1
13	Alert Condensable composite	Pentron	A2, A3, A3.5, B1, C2
Bulk Fill Base RBC			
14	Surefil SDR flow	Dentsply Sirona	Universal, A1, A2, A3
15	Filtek Bulk Fill Flowable	3M ESPE	Universal, A1, A2, A3
16	Venus Bulk Fill	Heraeus Kulzer	Universal
17	Tetric EvoFlow Bulk-Fill	Ivoclar-Vivadent	Universal shades IVA, IVB, IVW
18	X-tra base	VOCO	Universal, A2
19	QuiXX Posterior	Dentsply Sirona	Universal
20	Beautifil Bulk Flow GIOMER	SHOFU	Dentin, universal
21	Bulk Base Hard	MORITA	
22	Capo bulk fill plus	Schütz dental	Universal dentin colour natural appearance
23	Dexta fill bulk	Dexter	D, U
24	Estelite Bulk Fill Flow	Tokuyama Dental	U, B1, A1, A2, A3
25	EverX Flow	GC	Bulk shade, dentin shade
26	Geanial Bulk Injectable	GC	A1, A2
27	LC Base	Parkell	Universal
28	Palfique Bulk Flow	Tokuyama Dental	A1, A2, A3, B1, U
29	Opus Bulk Fill Flow	FGM	A1, A2, A3
Sonic activated bulk fill			

Table 2.1 (continued)

	Composite BF	Manufacturer	Shades available
30	SonicFill	Kerr	A1, A2, A3, B1
31	SonicFill 2	Kerr	A1, A2, A3, B1
32	Sonic fill 3	Kerr	A1, A2, A3
Thermo viscous technology			
33	VisCalor bulk	VOCO	U, A1, A2, A3
Dual cured bulk fill			
34	Fill Up!	Coltene-Whaledent	A2, A3
35	HyperFil	Parkell	A1, A2, B1, B2
36	Bulk EZ	Danville	A1, A2, A3
37	Bulk EZ PLUS	Zest dental solutions	A1, A2, A3, A3.5, B1, B2, B3, C2, C3, BL, OP, CORE WHITE
38	Profil Bulk Fill	Silmet	U, enamel
39	Light-core (fiber reinforced)	BISCO	Translucent and blue shades
40	N'Durance dimer Core	Septodont	Bleach white
41	ParaCore	Coltene/Whaledent	Dentin, white, translucent
42	Spee-Dee build up	Pulpdent	Yellow, white
43	Activa bioactive	Pulpdent	A1, A2, A3, A3.5
44	Admira fusion x-tra	VOCO	Omni-chromatic shade covers classic shade range
45	Bis-core (DC)	BISCO	Natural and opaque
46	Bisfil 2B (CC) Self-cure	BISCO	Universal, A3 and A3.5 shade
47	Bisfil II Self-cured	BISCO	Universal
48	Clearfil Core (CC)	Kuraray Noritake	Neutral colour shade
49	Clearfil DC Core Plus (DC)	Kuraray Noritake	White
50	Clearfil PhotoCore	Kuraray Noritake	Translucent
51	Core-Flo DC	BISCO	Natural/A1 and opaque white
52	Core-Flo DC Lite	BISCO	Natural/A1 and opaque white shades
53	Core Restore 2 (DC)	Kerr	Universal, white, blue, untinted
54	HardCore (DC)	Pulpdent	Off-white colour

2.2 Composition and Microstructure

A resin composite is mainly composed of an organic (resin matrix) and inorganic part (fillers) linked by a coupling agent (silane) [1, 7]. Bulk fill materials have similar chemical composition to the conventional RBCs with some variations, related to the filler particles and resin matrix that will be discussed later in this chapter. In general, the main monomers which form the resin matrix of most composites are present, such as the Bis-GMA, UDMA, TEGDMA, and EBPDMA with a moderate molecular weight. Yet, other monomers with lower viscosities have been added. These changes contribute to the "bulk" characteristic of bulk fill composites [8].

2.2.1 Organic Phase (Resin Matrix)

2.2.1.1 Conventional Composite Monomer

Composite formulations are described in details in the literature [9–11]. The organic phase includes different monomers, additives, and a curing system. Commercial dental composites are based on Bis-GMA (2.2-bis[4-(2-hydroxy-3-methacryloyloxy-propoxy) phenyl propane) monomer, commonly called Bis-glycidyl methacrylate. This resin has an aromatic structure in the central part of the molecule, causing much larger barriers to rotate around the bonds, and thus increasing its stiffness [9]. Their high molecular weight (512 g/mol) explains their lower polymerization shrinkage and less water sorption compared to other monomers [12]. However, high molecular monomers are very viscous and the use of a diluent or a viscosity controller is mandatory to achieve filler loading and a workable consistency [10].

2.2.1.2 Bulk Fill Monomer Modifications

The common characteristic to all bulk fill composites is their application and polymerization in layers of 4 mm and even 5 mm for some products. Several modifications have been made to the bulk fill formulations, in particular concerning the translucency, the use of a polymerization modulator and a specific photo initiator.

There is no generalized composition for all bulk fill as each product is manufacturer dependent. For instance, *Surefil SDR* flow (DENTSPLY/Caulk) contains a specific monomer; *UDMA* (dimethacrylate urethane). The manufacturers claim that it has a stress decreasing resin (SDR) technology from which it obtained its name. This provides superior molecule flexibility, therefore eluding polymerization stress during curing. *Filtek bulk fill* flowable (3 M ESPE) is based on a combination of four different monomers: *Bis-GMA*, *UDMA*, *Procrylat*, and *Bis-EMA*. The UDMA-based monomer has a high molecular weight of 849 g/mol, thus decreasing polymerization shrinkage [8]. This monomer is modified to include a photoactive group which the manufacturer refers to it as the *"polymerization modulator."* Polymerization shrinkage is reduced when the material is exposed to light, and the photoactive groups are cleaved. Simultaneously the oligomer chain breaks, which contains the stress while generating radicals that can promote more conversion and crosslinking of the material maintaining the polymerization rate or degree of conversion [13]. Additionally, the Procrylat monomer is responsible for more fluidity hence reducing polymerization stress.

2.2.2 Inorganic Phase (Fillers)

2.2.2.1 Conventional Composite Fillers

Filler particles are used to fill and reinforce the resin matrix. They also improve the mechanical properties, provide radiopacity, minimize the coefficient of thermal expansion and are thought to reduce the polymerization shrinkage. The particle size will influence other properties such as surface roughness, polishability, and fluidity [11, 14].

Composites contain a variety of fillers such as fused silica (SiO_2), quartz, and radiopaque particles based on oxides of barium, strontium, zirconium, and other metals [12, 14]. Composite classifications are often based on their filler size, shape, and distribution. Size varies between 0.01 μm and 85 μm. Filler morphologies depends on the development process. Filler loading is expressed in percentages by weight or volume. In general, filler load ranges between 35 and 70 vol% or 50 and 85 wt% [15, 16].

Hybrid resin composites contain a heterogeneous aggregate of filler particles. They have a filler load of 70–80% by weight, with their size ranging from 0.04 μm and 1–5 μm. The average particle size of hybrid composites is usually >1 μm. This mixture of fillers gives them their excellent physical properties and high polishability, however, they are unable to maintain their gloss. Further refinements in the particle size resulted in composites with particles averaging about 0.4–1.0 μm which are referred to as "microhybrids." They may contain up to 60–70% of fillers by volume. These materials are generally considered to be universal composites as they can be used in both anterior and posterior cavities. Nowadays, the hybrid category represents the most used resin composite. A decade ago, nanofilled composites or nanohybrids were introduced onto the dental market. Those composites use nanoparticles ranging from 0.005 to 1 μm or 5–100 nm. They are linked together into what is called a ″nanocluster″ and are assumed to produce a composite restoration that has strength similar to hybrid composites yet smoother surfaces with high lustre resulting in optimal aesthetics. Nano fill describes filler particle sizes that have been used in microfill composites. The nanofilled composites present similar mechanical and physical properties to microhybrid composites, but polishability and gloss retention similar to micro filled composites [17].

2.2.2.2 Bulk Fill Filler Modifications

The percentage of fillers in bulk fill composite is 66–70% by volume and is lower than conventional microhybrid and nanohybrid composites. However, it has comparable percentage by volume to conventional flowable RBCs but higher percentage by weight. This can be explained by the large filler size (20 μm). The lower percentage of fillers with a bigger size, decreased the refractive index between the matrix and filler system, consequently permitting more light penetration, hence an increased depth of cure [8]. Manufacturers have identified many of the bulk fill components that improved the depth of cure, yet, some information remains undisclosed such as the ratio of each monomer, the filler content or their proprietary formulations.

For example, Tetric N-Ceram Bulk fill (TBF; Ivoclar Vivadent, Schaan, Liechtenstein) and SDR (Caulk DENTSPLY, York, PA, USA) were launched with the manufacturer claiming that they contain a *shrinkage stress reliever* that minimizes polymerization shrinkage [18].

2.2.3 Microstructure

A study that evaluated the polymerization performance and depth of cure of highly filled conventional flowable and bulk fill resin composites it has been shown that the composition affected the linear polymerization shrinkage and polymerization shrinkage stress measurement [18]. Rafaela A. Melo et al. evaluated the chemical composition and other parameters of a regular high viscosity bulk fill and a traditional composite resin. They prepared 80 samples of (Aura/SDI, FiltekZ250 XT/3 M, Aura Bulk Fill/SDI, and Filtek Bulk Fill/3 M). Scanning electron microscopy (SEM) and energy dispersity spectroscopy (EDS) were used to assess the morphology of the filler particles present and the chemical characteristics of the composites. They found that the elements carbon, oxygen, silicon, and aluminium were present in all composites studied. In addition to those elements barium and zirconia were found in Aura bulk fill. Zirconia was also found in large amounts in Filtek bulk fill and fluoride. Two other studies of bulk fill composition found similar inorganic elements in various amounts including silicon, aluminium, fluoride, barium, and zirconia. The purpose of adding those specific elements was to improve optical density properties of the composite including other properties [19].

Differences in filler content and the SEM are given in Table 2.2.

Table 2.2 Comparison between some conventional composites and bulk fill resin composites from the same manufacturer

Manufacturer	Material	Composition	Filler loading	Filler's morphology (SEM) 10.00 Kx
3MESPE	Filtek Z350 XT	UDMA, Bis-GMA, TEGDMA	55.6 vol% 72.5 wt%	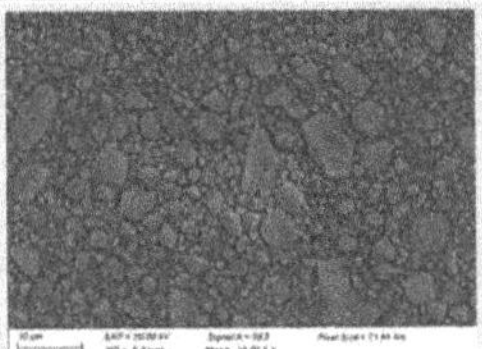
	Filtek One Bulk Fill	AUDMA), UDMA, addition fragmentation 1, 12-dodecane-DMA	76.5 wt% 58.4 vol%	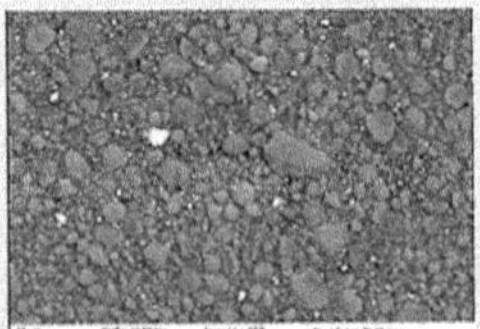
Kavo Kerr	Harmonize	Bis-GMA UDMA TEGDMA Bis-EMA6	78.5 wt% 63.3 vol%	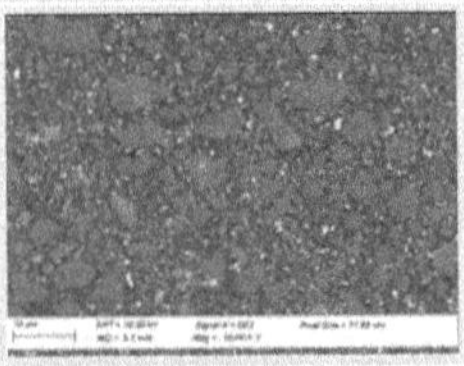
	Sonic fill	Bis-GMA TEGDMA Bis-EMA	83.5 wt%	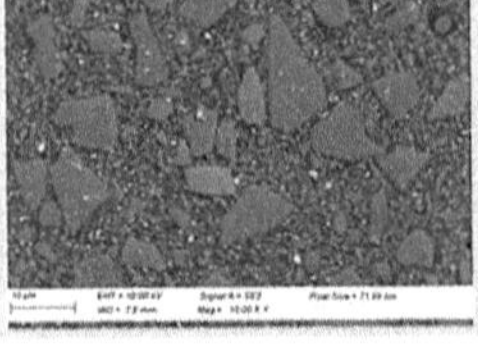

Table 2.2 (continued)

Manufacturer	Material	Composition	Filler loading	Filler's morphology (SEM) 10.00 K×
Voco	GrandioSO	Bis-GMA, Bis-EMA, TEGDMA	89 wt%	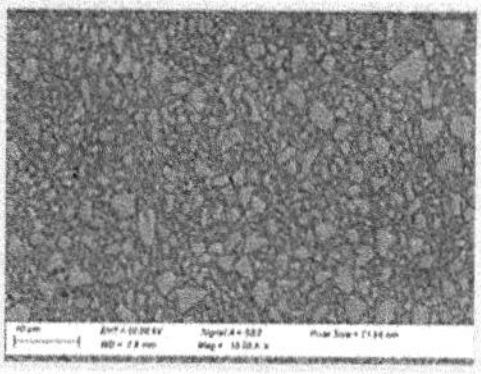
	Grandioso Flow	Bis-EMA MMA	80% wt	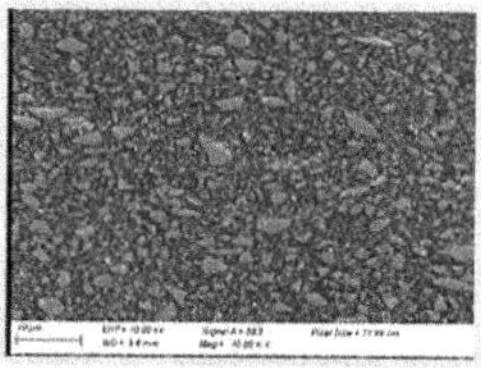
GC	Geanial Universal Flow	UDMA, TEGDMA, Bis-MEPP, silicon dioxide, strontium glass	50 vol% 69 wt%	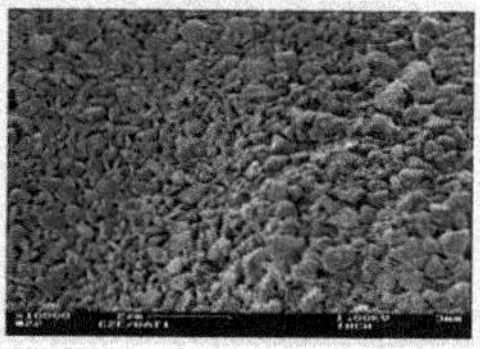
	EverX posterior	Bis-GMA TEGDMA PMMA	53.6 vol%	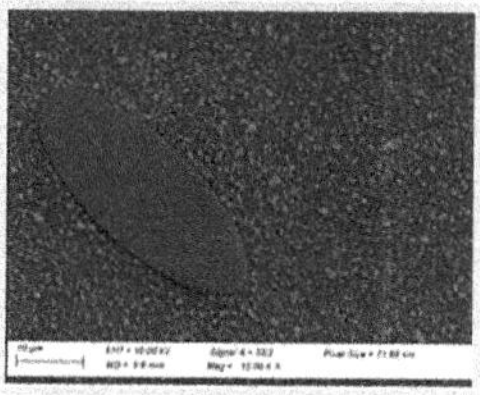
Ivoclar	Tetric Evoceram Bulk fill	Bis-GMA UDMA Bis-EMA	80 wt% 61 vol% Barium glass filler	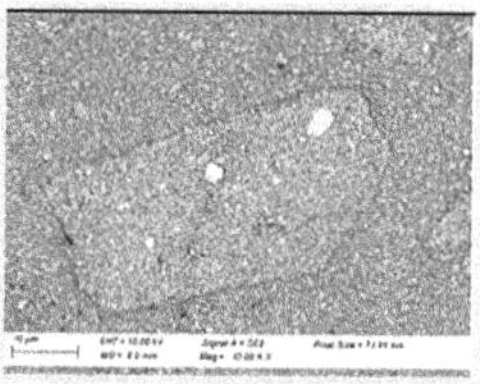
	Tetric Power fill	Bis-GMA, Bis-EMA, UDMA, Bis-PMA, DCP, D3MA	(79 wt%, 53–54 vol%) Barium glass, ytterbium, Trifluoride, copolymer, mixed oxide (SiO_2/ZrO_2)	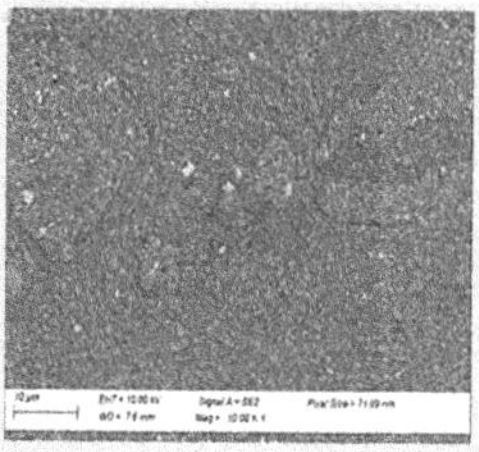

SEM photomicrographs of the fillers at 10,000× magnification are shown in Fig. 2.1a–f. Filler size included both small or large fillers, while their shapes included angular, rounded or spherical, depending on the product. Different shapes of fillers were observed for the materials of the same category.

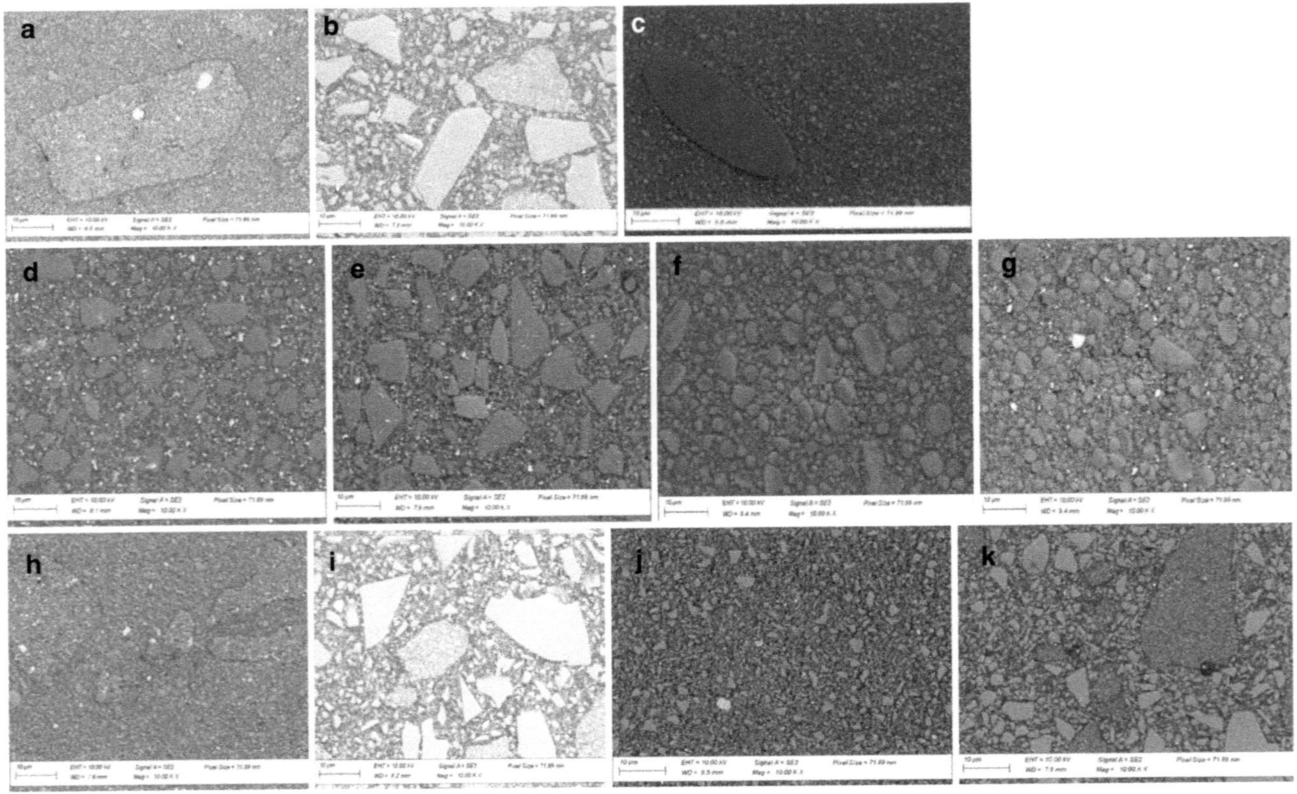

Fig. 2.1 The SEM photomicrographs above (**a**–**f**) are of the fillers at 10,000× magnification show filler morphology of some pairs of resin composites (conventional versus bulk fill resin composites), (**a**) Tetric EvoCeram Bulk fill (**b**)Tetric EvoFlow Bulk fill (**c**) EverX posterior (**d**) Harmonize (**e**) SonicFill 3 (**f**) Filtek Supreme XTE (**g**) one Bulk Fill (**h**) Tetric PowerFill (**i**) Tetric Power Flow (**j**) Venus Bulk fill (**k**) Beautifil

Some pairs of resin composites issued from the same manufacturer (universal versus a flowable of highly filled bulk) were compared (a) Tetric EvoCeram Bulk fill (b)Tetric EvoFlow Bulk (d) Harmonize and (e) Sonicfill 3, (f) Filtek Supreme XTE (g) one Bulk Fill, (h) Tetric PowerFill, (i) Tetric Power Flow.

For each pair of composites, at least one feature, the shape or the percentage of fillers or the composition of the organic matrix was modified. Some bulk fill resin composites showed bigger fillers size like Sonicfill 3 (e), Tetric Power Flow (i), and Beautiful (k), while others showed similar size to their corresponding conventional from the same manufacturer, Harmonize (d) and Sonicfill (e) and Filtek Supreme XTE (g) one Bulk Fill.

2.2.4 Coupling Agent (Silanes)

As the two major constituents of resin composites are chemically different, the bond between the inorganic fillers and resin matrix is provided for by the coupling agent or silane. Coupling agents work better with silica particles. Therefore, most of dental composites are based on silica-containing fillers [14]. The most common used coupling agent is the MPMA (γ-methacryloxypropyl-trimethoxy silane) followed by APM (γ-acryloxypropyl-trimethoxysilane). It has been shown that the presence of silane enhances the mechanical properties of resin composites and protects the filler surfaces [20]. The presence of silane allows greater filler loading, thus reducing the polymerization shrinkage. Nevertheless, the interfaces between filler particles and the matrix are the weakest link and may be destroyed by hydrolytic degradation [21]. A bond failure can occur at the silane–filler interface, resulting in a filler debonding with leaching of the monomers [22, 23]. In order to improve filler-matrix coupling and to enhance wear and fatigue-resistance of resin composites, chemical decontamination methods are employed as pre-treatment of the silanization process [24]. Various cleaning processes are reported in the literature, including the use of acids, bases, and organic solvents at several temperatures.

2.2.4.1 Polymerization Initiation System of Bulk Fill

Some manufacturers have added novel photo initiator such as Ivocerin, by Ivoclar vivadent in Tetric Evoceram bulk fill. This photo initiator acts as a polymerization promoter that is based on the chemical element Ge (germanium), which makes Ivocerin more reactive due to greater absorption of 400–450 nm when compared to the traditional photo initiator camphorquinone. It has been claimed that it also can filter light pollution, giving a more suitable clinical working time [8].

2.3 Classification of Bulk Fill Composite

The exact composition of many of the currently available bulk fill materials is not made available by the manufacturers making it impossible to develop an accurate classification of the materials [25]. They can be categorized according to their viscosity and mode of application (Fig. 2.2).

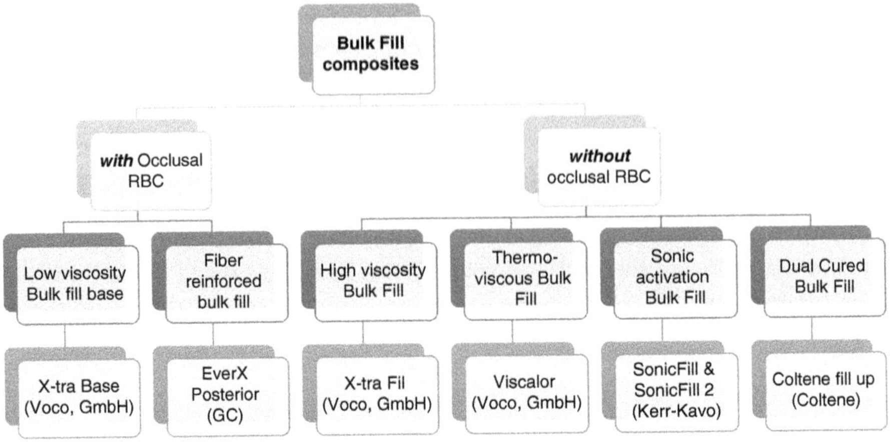

Fig. 2.2 Bulk fill composite classification

2.3.1 According to Viscosity

2.3.1.1 Low Viscosity Bulk Fill

A base bulk fill is a low viscosity flowable material facilitating placement through a small nozzle of a syringe. This helps in their adaptation in deeper and less accessible cavities. They display inferior mechanical properties; the surface is less wear resistance due to the lower amount of fillers present compared to conventional/microhybrid or nanohybrid resin composites. Thus, overlaying with a conventional composite is necessary, representing a two-step bulk fill technique. These base bulk fills are also named flowable bulk fill composites [25–28].

2.3.1.2 High Viscosity Bulk Fill

The full body bulk fill composites have a higher inorganic filler content when compared to the low viscosity base bulk fills, causing them to be more wear resistant and better at handling masticatory load. Hence, they can be used to fill all of the cavity and sculpt its occlusal surface as a final layer without the need to be covered with a conventional composite. This group of bulk fills are a true representation of the bulk fill category allowing the reconstruction of the lost tooth structures [25, 28, 29].

2.3.2 Modified High Viscosity Bulk Fill

2.3.2.1 Sonically Activated Bulk Fill

The high viscosity bulk fills have better mechanical properties when compared to the low viscosity bulk fills, whereas, the low viscosity base bulk fills are easier to apply into deeper cavities. Sonic activated bulk fill material (SonicFill and SonicFill 2, and more recently SonicFill 3 Kerr; Orange, CA, USA) have been introduced. These are high viscosity bulk fill which are dispensed via an air-driven hand piece using sonic vibration resulting in a reduction in the materials viscosity by almost 84%. As a result it can be applied easily into the cavity as a flowable composite, before resuming to its more viscous state which can then be sculped in the required anatomy [25, 28, 30].

2.3.2.2 Thermo-Viscous Bulk Fill

VisCalor bulk fill is the first material on the market that uses thermo-viscous-technology. The filler surface is treated and synchronized with the resin matrix which aids in prolongation of its reduced viscosity during the increase in temperature. The effect of this technology is a material that is applied in a flowable consistency at a temperature of 68 °C via a composite warmer or the new VisCalor dispenser, yet it is sculpatable like packable composites at normal temperature.

2.3.2.3 Fibre-Reinforced Bulk Fill

There are other high viscosity composites, which can be placed in bulk; they contain glass fibre fillers that reinforce the tooth/composite complex when restored. These include EverX Posterior (GC). These fibre-reinforced composites are used as a dentine substitute when restoring large cavities. The fibre fillers tend to prevent and inhibit crack propagation, avoiding fracture which is one of the most common reasons for composite failure [25].

2.3.3 Dual Cured Bulk Fill Composite Resin

Bulk fill composites can be also categorized according to their photo polymerization mode; light or dual-cure bulk fill composites [31, 32]. The dual cured BFC such as fill-up have a low filler load (65% Wt.), yet manufacturers state that this material can be used without a conventional RBC as a final layer. Due to the lack of clinical studies to support this information, authors alert clinicians, that low filler content in composite would be expected to make it less wear resistant [28].

2.3.4 Clinical Relevance

The mechanical characteristics of bulk fill composites vary based on the quantity of inorganic fillers present. Hence, low viscosity materials which exhibit low wear resistance require an additional cap layer of conventional composite. In addition to the occlusal surfaces, authors advice that proximal contact points be restored with conventional composite when using low viscosity base bulk fills due to the risk of wear alongside the adjacent tooth leading to an open contact [28, 33]. Furthermore, another reason for covering the bulk fill composite with acceptable wear resistance is aesthetic as many BFs are translucent. Some base bulk fills have a similar filler content to high viscosity materials, whereas some high viscosity bulk fills have mechanical characteristics comparable to the low viscosity BF, making the decision to use a specific material more difficult [34]. In general, all of the bulk fill composites could be covered with a conventional resin composite, to enhance both aesthetics and their physical properties [28]. For example, SDR which is a flowable BF requires a conventional composite resin layer on top of it.

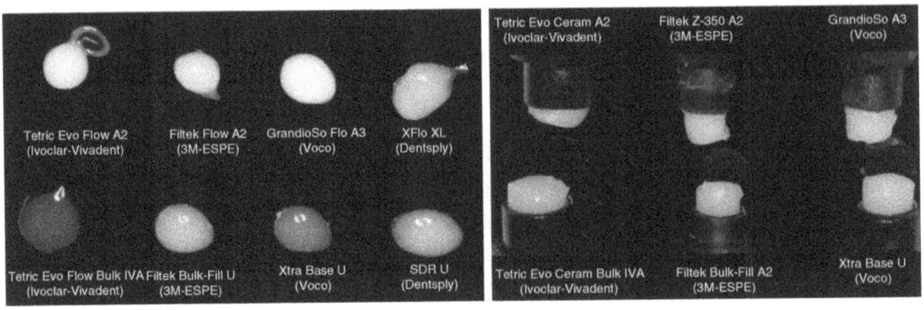

Fig. 2.3 Comparison of bulk fill shades to conventional composite

2.4 Bulk Fill Shades and Depth of Cure

Every manufacturing company provide their own shades for bulk fill composites. However, the shades tend to be more translucent than similar shades of conventional universal composites as displayed in Fig. 2.3.

Translucency is an optical characteristic that is highly distinct in bulk fill composites, when compared to conventional composites. This property is affected by several parameters such as the size and percentage of fillers, translucency of fillers, opacifiers, organic resin, and refractive index of the resin. When the refractive index of the resin and organic fillers is almost the same the material is more translucent.

The high translucency facilitates the penetration of light through the resin during polymerization increasing the degree of conversion and depth of cure. This explains the ability of bulk fill to be placed in an increment of more than 4 mm. Low viscosity bulk fill composites have a low filler load making the composite more translucent, hence a greater depth of cure. Despite their better DOC, other properties are compromised to obtain this translucency, such as aesthetics. If aesthetics is a priority for patient in posterior region, a capping layer of conventional composite can be placed as it is compatible with most bulk fill materials. Some manufacturers have tried to eliminate this limitation, such as Ivoclar by introducing "*asencio*" the chameleon effect bulk fill which increases in opacity post polymerization. Also the SonicFill (Kerr) which can be applied in a single layer technique [7, 13, 28].

Acknowledgments The authors would like to express sincere gratitude to Dr. Hamad Algamaiah for providing SEM fillers images.

References

1. Ferracane JL. Resin composite—state of the art. Dent Mater. 2011;27(1):29–38.
2. Rasines Alcaraz MG, Veitz-Keenan A, Sahrmann P, Schmidlin PR, Davis D, Iheozor-Ejiofor Z. Direct composite resin fillings versus amalgam fillings for permanent or adult posterior teeth. Cochrane Database Syst Rev. 2014;31(3):CD005620.

3. Schricker SR. Composite resin polymerization and relevant parameters. In: Eliades T, Brantley WA, editors. Orthodontic applications of biomaterials. Cambridge: Woodhead Publishing; 2017. p. 153–70.
4. Weinmann W, Thalacker C, Fau-Guggenberger R, Guggenberger R. Siloranes in dental composites. Dent Mater. 2005;21:68–74.
5. Mantri SP, Mantri SS. Management of shrinkage stresses in direct restorative light-cured composites: a review. J Esthet Restor Dent. 2013;25(5):305–13.
6. Leinfelder KF. Posterior composite resins. J Am Dent Assoc. 1988;117(4):21E–6E.
7. Sabbagh J, Hajj M, Feghali M, Mansour H. Les composites en monocouche ou bulk-fill partie I-composition, particularités et classification. Biomatériaux Cliniques. 2016;2:12–8.
8. Corral-Núnez C, Vildósola-Grez P, Bersezio-Miranda C, Alves-Dos Campos E, Fernández GE. State of the art of bulk-fill resin-based composites: a review. Rev Fac Odontol Univ Antioq. 2015;27(1):177–96.
9. Peutzfeldt A. Resin composites in dentistry: the monomer systems. Eur J Oral Sci. 1997;105(2):97–116.
10. Moszner N, Salz U. New developments of polymeric dental composites. Prog Polym Sci. 2001;26(4):535–76.
11. Braden M, Clarke RL, Parker S, Nicholson J. Polymeric dental materials. Berlin: Springer Science & Business Media; 1997.
12. Albers HF. Tooth-colored restoratives: principles and techniques. Toronto, ON: BC Decker; 2002.
13. Fugolin APP, Pfeifer CS. New resins for dental composites. J Dent Res. 2017;96(10):1085–91.
14. Ritter AV, Boushell LW, Walter R. Sturdevant's art and science of operative dentistry. 7th ed. St. Louis: Elsevier; 2019.
15. Anusavice KJ, Shen C, Rawls HR. Phillips science of dental materials. 12th ed. Philadelphia: Saunders; 2003.
16. Sabbagh J, Bachérius L, Biebuyck JJ, Vreven J, Lambrechts P, Leloup G. Characterization of the inorganic fraction of resin composites. J Oral Rehabil. 2004;31(11):1090–101.
17. Tuncer S, Demirci M, Öztaş E, Tekçe N, Uysal Ö. Microhybrid versus nanofill composite in combination with a three step etch and rinse adhesive in occlusal cavities: five year results. Restor Dent Endod. 2017;42(4):253–63.
18. Jang JH, Park SH, Hwang IN. Polymerization shrinkage and depth of cure of bulk-fill resin composites and highly filled flsowable resin. Oper Dent. 2015;40(2):172–80.
19. Melo RA, Bispo ASL, Barbosa GAS, Galvão MR, de Assunção IV, Souza ROA, et al. Morphochemical characterization, microhardness, water sorption, and solubility of regular viscosity bulk fill and traditional composite resins. Microsc Res Tech. 2019;82(9):1500–6.
20. Mohsen NM, Craig RG. Hydrolytic stability of silanated zirconia-silica-urethane dimethacrylate composites. J Oral Rehabil. 1995;22(3):213–20.
21. Santerre JP, Shajii L, Leung BW. Relation of dental composite formulations to their degradation and the release of hydrolyzed polymeric-resin-derived products. Crit Rev Oral Biol Med. 2001;12(2):136–51.
22. Calais JG, Soderholm KJM. Influence of filler type and water exposure on flexural strength of experimental composite resins. J Dent Res. 1988;67(5):836–40.
23. Spahl W, Budzikiewicz H, Geurtsen W. Determination of leachable components from four commercial dental composites by gas and liquid chromatography/mass spectrometry. J Dent. 1998;26(2):137–45.
24. Shirai K, Yoshida Y, Nakayama Y, Fujitani M, Shintani H, Wakasa K, et al. Assessment of decontamination methods as pretreatment of silanization of composite glass fillers. J Biomed Mater Res. 2000;53(3):204–10.
25. Van Ende A, De Munck J, Lise DP, Van Meerbeek B, Ermis B. Bulk-fill composites: a review of the current literature. J Adhes Dent. 2017;19(2):95–109.
26. Al-Nabulsi M, Daud A, Yiu C, Omar H, Sauro S, Fawzy A, et al. Co-blend application mode of bulk fill composite resin. Materials (Basel). 2019;12:122504.

27. Kaptan A. Bulk fill composites. J Dent Oral Health. 2019; 1.
28. Chesterman J, Jowett A, Gallacher A, Nixon P. Bulk-fill resin-based composite restorative materials: a review. Br Dent J. 2017;222(5):337–44.
29. Veloso SRM, Lemos CAA, de Moraes SLD, do Egito Vasconcelos BC, Pellizzer EP, de Melo Monteiro GQ. Clinical performance of bulk-fill and conventional resin composite restorations in posterior teeth: a systematic review and meta-analysis. Clin Oral Investig. 2019;23(1):221–33.
30. Reis AF, Vestphal M, Amaral RC, Rodrigues JA, Roulet J-F, Roscoe MG. Efficiency of polymerization of bulk-fill composite resins: a systematic review. Braz Oral Res. 2017;31:e59.
31. Aggarwal N, Jain A, Gupta H, Abrol A, Singh C, Rapgay T. The comparative evaluation of depth of cure of bulk-fill composites invitro study. J Conserv Dent. 2019;22(4):371–5.
32. Lima RBW, Troconis CCM, Moreno MBP, Murillo-Gómez F, De Goes MF. Depth of cure of bulk fill resin composites: a systematic review. J Esthet Restor Dent. 2018;30(6):492–501.
33. Al-Nahedh HN, Alawami Z. Fracture resistance and marginal adaptation of capped and uncapped bulk-fill resin-based materials. Oper Dent. 2020;45(2):E43–56.
34. Haugen HJ, Marovic D, Par M, Khai Le Thieu M, Reseland JE, Johnsen GF. Bulk fill composites have similar performance to conventional dental composites. Int J Mol Sci. 2020;21(14):5136.

Bulk Fill Composites: Adhesion and Interfacial Adaptation

3

Alireza Sadr, Omri Margalit, Alexander Palander, and Junji Tagami

3.1 The Evolution of Adhesives

Historically both composite polymers and metal restorations relied on mechanical retention to tooth structure. This technique required the practitioner to remove large amounts of affected and even sound tooth structure. Retention forms were more invasive, and yielded poor results in terms of biocompatibility, aesthetics, and efficacy. These non-adhesive restorations also created a potential gap at the interface of composite and hard tissue, which was susceptible to leakage, demineralization, and secondary caries. Issues derived from the mechanical retention practice ultimately led to restoration failure and filling dislodgement. The advent of adhesive dentistry addressed these barriers and simultaneously adopted a minimally invasive approach.

Adhesive dentistry is the conservative practice of using resin-based materials bonded directly to tooth structure. This preserves uncompromised hard tissues, eliminates mechanical retention, and improves the marginal seal of composite fillings.

A. Sadr (✉)
Biomimetics Biomaterials Biophotonics Biomechanics and Technology Laboratory, Department of Restorative Dentistry, University of Washington, Seattle, WA, USA

Cariology and Operative Dentistry Department, Graduate School of Medical and Dental Sciences, Tokyo Medical and Dental University, Tokyo, Japan
e-mail: arsadr@uw.edu

O. Margalit · A. Palander
Biomimetics Biomaterials Biophotonics Biomechanics and Technology Laboratory, Department of Restorative Dentistry, University of Washington, Seattle, WA, USA
e-mail: omrimar@uw.edu; apalander@uw.edu

J. Tagami
Cariology and Operative Dentistry Department, Graduate School of Medical and Dental Sciences, Tokyo Medical and Dental University, Tokyo, Japan
e-mail: Tagami.ope@tmd.ac.jp

J. Sabbagh, R. McConnell (eds.), *Bulk Fill Resin Composites in Dentistry*,
https://doi.org/10.1007/978-3-031-16388-3_3

3.1.1 The Acid Etch Technique and Early Dentin Bond

Enamel bonding was initially achieved in the 1950s with penetration of resin monomer to acid-etched enamel [1]. The etching approach only was sufficient for bonding to enamel but bonding to dentin was significantly more challenging due to its organic composition and inhomogeneous deposition. Recall that enamel is approximately 90% hydroxyapatite crystals (mineral content) in the form of parallel enamel prisms and interrod enamel. Dentin on the other hand is a complex organic matrix of odontoblasts, type I collagen, mineral and fluid filled microchannel dentinal tubules. The water and hydrophilic composition of dentin repelled the hydrophobic resins from penetrating deep into the dentin. This meant that with acid-etch technique resin was not impregnating deep enough for the micromechanical retention.

Bonding to dentin was eventually achieved by Fusayama, who pioneered the "total-etch" (also called "etch-and-rinse") technique [2]. This process was most noteworthy for removing the smear layer created by instrumentation. This was achieved through chelating excess metal and mineral from the preparation surface. Though it may seem trivial, the smear layer occluded the dentinal tubules and directly inhibited primer or bond from impregnating fully into the dentin. Fusayama found that demineralizing the dentin with 30–40% acid also exposed the collagen fibrils which could then be used to integrate and copolymerize a hydrophilic monomer. Demineralization of dentin to 3–5 μm created ideal pores or voids that are filled by primer/resin for micromechanical retention.

Traditionally, the term of adhesion to dentin referred to the three-step process of etching, priming, and bonding adhesive resin into a tooth surface. Adhesive bonds use micromechanical retention, which is achieved through acid etching and priming underlying tooth structure. These steps allow adhesive resin to integrate into the porous surface of prepared tooth structure, rather than polymerizing on the surface of the preparation. Etching is the application of phosphoric acid (H_3PO_4) or a similar strong acid to demineralize the bonding surface. Exposed projections of hydroxyapatite increase the surface area to bond to and are more receptive to diffusion of hydrophobic resin. When polymerized, monomers of the adhesive resin interlock with these extensions. Priming is the step that removes excess water and expands the collagen network to allow for better wettability by the adhesive. Preparing the bonding surface for bond in this way is not as vital for an etched and dried enamel, but is very important for bonding to dentin. Finally, the bond is worked into the extensions of the prep and light cured to lock into the prepared microenvironment. It is this final layer that links the composite filling material to the tooth surface. Without adhesive bonds, composite restorations are just retentive resin fillings and have failures associated with an incomplete marginal seal and gap formation. OptiBond FL (Kerr, Brea, CA) has shown a record of accomplishment of success over decades after its introduction [1].

The mechanism for this loss of integrity was hydrolytic dissolution of both the polymer and the demineralized tissue (collagen fibrils). The organic component of dentin was left unprotected at sites of incomplete infiltration of resin, a process known as nanoleakage. Dentinal collagen is susceptible to hydrolytic cleavage in water, as well as attack from host-derived enzymes such as matrix metalloproteases

(MMPs). To remedy this, researchers sought resins that promoted chemical interaction and provided an impermeable interface with the tooth substrate.

The advent of etch-and-rinse technique solved the issues associated with penetrating the smear layer for dentinal bonding. However, there was still hydrophilic and organic substances within the microcosm of the preparation surface that would not mix well with hydrophobic resin. Hydrophobicity is important for bonding agents to inhibit degradation in the oral environment. Thus, an adhesive needed to integrate the hydrophilic natural dentin structure with the hydrophobic adhesive monomers. It is the role of the primer to accomplish this necessary component of dental bonding. The primer acts to: (1) remove water and (2) chemically interact with collagen and hydroxyapatite. Removing excess water is accomplished through evaporation, which the primers can promote with polar solvents, mainly acetone. Primers also contain water, ethanol or acetone to decrease viscosity during the initial application, which helps the primer flow into all areas of the preparation. In addition, a successful primer contains substrates that can chemically attract both the hydrophobic resin and the hydrophilic tooth. Lastly, the literature supports mechanical stimulation of the primer by the practitioner at the time of application. In conjunction with etch-and-rinse, primers allow for adhesive polymerization to interlock the resin and the tooth structure intimately. The hydrophobic resin is the final component (and layer) to the three-step procedure of bonding. Monomer entanglement with collagen fibrils creates a mixed structure at the resin-dentin interface is known as the "hybrid layer," as coined by Nakabayashi. After curing, this final mixture of primer, resin, and etched tooth extensions at the margin of a preparation creates an impermeable seal.

3.1.2 The Single-Bottle Adhesive and Wet Bonding

As technology sought to increase efficiency, manufacturers tried to conserve the number of steps required for proper bonding technique. In the fourth-generation system, the first operator coats H_3PO_4 on all prepared surfaces; this is the "total etch" or "etch and rinse" technique. After rinsing, a primer is used that allows the collagen fibers in the tooth to take on a more suitable spatial organization. Drying is important to allow volatile solvents to evaporate off excess water at this time. A third and final step is the application of bond, which integrates into the prepped collagen fibers. The attempt to simplify adhesive steps resulted in fifth generation of adhesives, which is a two-step system; etchant is the first step as before, and the second step includes a primer and bond in the same solution. The challenge was to keep the dentin wet enough to prevent the collapse of the collagen after phosphoric acid etching but not to leave too much moisture (visible water droplets) that would hamper effective polymerization. The term "wet-bonding" technique described this challenge for the fifth generation adhesives. Research showed that penetration of these single-bottle adhesives "two-step etch-and-rinse" into dentin was more challenging than originally thought, with areas of incompletely impregnated collagen at the base of hybrid layer, increasing the chance for long-term degradation of the bond and leakage.

3.1.3 The Self-Etch Approach

Development of the functional acidic monomer played a pivotal role in the introduction of clinically effective self-etching adhesives. One of the most successful acidic monomers in the composition of self-etch systems is 10-methacryloxydecyl dihydrogen phosphate (MDP) originally developed by Kuraray Noritake Dental, Tokyo, Japan. This monomer has a C=C bond on one end for polymerization and a reactive acidic moiety on the other end. The concept of chemical bonding to apatite gained strength by the observations of Van Meerbeek et al. on the self-orientation of the MDP monomer when reacting with the apatite, termed nanolayering. Electron microscopic observation of the interface between an MDP-containing two-step self-etch system, Clearfil SE Bond (Kuraray) and dentin after acid-base challenge showed that the self-etch adhesive system demineralized dentin mildly and partially, leaving hydroxyapatite crystals in the base of the hybrid layer. The phosphoric acid moiety in MDP could form an insoluble salt with the calcium-rich apatite, thereby forming a stable bond. The sixth generation adhesive, two-step self-etch, uses a self-etching primer in the first step, and a pure resin bond applied in the last [3].

Seventh generation relies on an all-in-one solution where all three components: etchant, primer, and bond are within one product. The all-in-one adhesives developed further to include additional components such as silane coupling agents for ceramic bonding and hydrophilic components facilitating penetration of the adhesive into etched dentin. This allowed more versatility, and the clinicians could choose a total-etching technique followed by application of the universal adhesive. The etching of dentin is an option open to the clinicians for these universal self-etch adhesives; however, they generally have a higher pH to improve their shelf-life stability, which means they are less effectiveness in enamel etching. Therefore, a selective enamel etching step is highly recommended for these generation systems by etching the enamel alone [4]. This step is particularly important, since the debonding at external margins has been typically considered more important than the internal dentin interface gaps, due to the increased risk of discoloration, bacterial leakage, and formation of caries around open margins [5]. While the dentin bond strength values are similar between the phosphoric acid-etching and self-etching of dentin with universal adhesives across studies [6, 7] Some have advised against etching of the dentin and particularly the dentin-enamel junction (DEJ) zone, due to the increased risk of hydrolytic degradation of hybrid layer and undermined cohesive strength of the DEJ [8, 9].

Self-adhesive bulk-fill restorative are the latest introduction in this category. These materials are mainly developed based on a combination of functional adhesive monomer technologies and bulk-fill composites through polymerizable acid polymers [10]. While promising, at the time, there is no evidence on the long-term clinical success of these materials. Historically, the bond strengths obtained with self-adhesive composites and glass-ionomer family of products have been inferior to those of multi-step adhesives, simply due to the fact that sufficient penetration of monomers in a liquid form is considered crucial for successful bonding (Fig. 3.1).

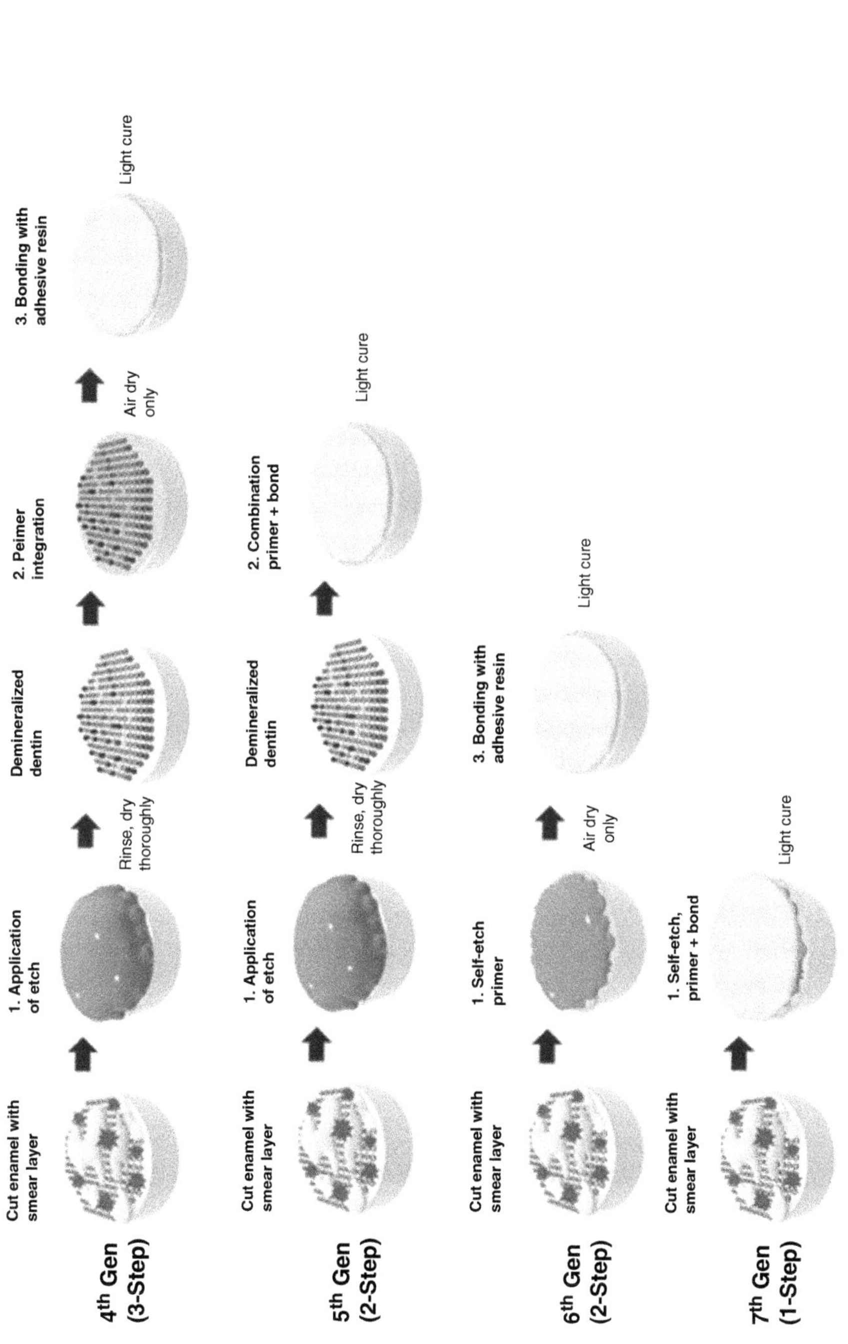

Fig. 3.1 Bond generation 4–7. Note that in the combination self-etching techniques of generations 6 and 7, the smear layer is not removed, but penetrated by the combination etch + primer

3.2 Bonding Implications for Bulk Fill Composites

Creating a sound bond to tooth structure important for any composite restoration, and clinicians should be reminded of the implications of adhesives for the bulk-fill technique. The most notable subject is shrinkage stress, accounting for a number of issues when attempting the bulk fill technique.

Polymerization shrinkage is a decrease in volume as methacrylate composite monomer is converted into polymer. This decrease in entropy creates a force that disrupts the adhesive hybrid layer that the clinician worked so hard to establish. Shrinkage stress may pull adhesive from the margin to ruin micromechanical retention. The shrinkage force causes fractures within the composite, adhesive and even the remaining sound tooth structure, known as a cohesive fault. Fractures allow for bacterial leakage, which can lead to demineralization and secondary caries. Additionally, when the composite restoration is placed under masticatory forces and thermal stress, a compromised margin can lead to even further damage (A). Polymerization can also lead to measurable gap formation at the pulpal floor of cavity preparations, contributing to a loss of marginal seal. These occurrences are observed as a direct result of shrinkage, but the bulk-fill technique alone is not to blame, obtaining proper adhesion is key.

Gap formation and loss of marginal seal is linked to the direction of polymerization shrinkage, and not only the size of the restoration. That is, polymerization from the outer most or occlusal/coronal surfaces toward the pulpal extensions of the prep will lead to the composite pulling inward and off the pulpal floor or away from the preparation walls. This is seen in vitro as measurable gaps and loss of margins. In contrast, polymerization shrinkage that originates at the margins of the restoration will result in shrinkage at the outermost layer, pulling composite into the preparation. The latter direction is the beneficial result of shrinkage that eliminates the issues associated with marginal seal and gap formation. In trying to standardize shrinkage to achieve this desirable direction, it was thought that the origin of the light source (occlusal versus marginal) was key. However, Versluis determined that the direction of shrinkage was mostly determined by the quality of the bond to the tooth and presence of unbonded surfaces [11]. Thus, it is advised that clinicians who are trying to create clinically acceptable results should appreciate the importance of adhesion and manage the polymerization shrinkage stress when placing large restorations.

3.3 What Adhesive Strategy Should Work for Bulk Fill Composites?

With the challenges of the bulk fill strategy, selection of the bonding system is an important step for a successful restoration. It is important to create adequate and timely copolymerization between the adhesive layer and the bulk fill composite to resist the competition between shrinkage stress development and maturing dentin bond.

From a clinical chair time management point of view, it makes sense to combine a bulk filling approach with a single-step all-in-one or universal adhesive. This offers a simplified application procedure resulting in reduced chair time compared with the two-step self-etching adhesives that required at least two separate application steps. While most of these bonding systems have reached comparable bond strength values to the tooth structure under laboratory conditions, the performance of the simplified adhesives has been questioned due to concerns regarding inherent limitations of their chemical mix of hydrophobic and hydrophilic components [12]. The water-free hydrophobic bonding agent of the two-step approach could slow down the hydrolytic degradation of the hybrid layer and contribute to tight sealing [13].

The real-time imaging of one-step and two-step self-etch adhesives when a flowable composite was bulk-filled showed that in the former, the separation mainly occurred only 7–14 s after the light curing started [14]. It is noteworthy that under that study, composite polymerization developed slower in deeper areas. Therefore, the dentin gap formation at the deeper cavity interface seemed to have occurred when the shallower composite had reached the postgel phase. Those findings also demonstrated that new polymerization shrinkage-related gaps were unlikely to initiate after the 20-s light-curing period; however, the propagation of existing defects evidently continued in a logarithmic pattern in the few minutes following completion of the light irradiation, as the postgel shrinkage continued in the composite despite the expected relaxation of residual stress [14] (Fig. 3.2).

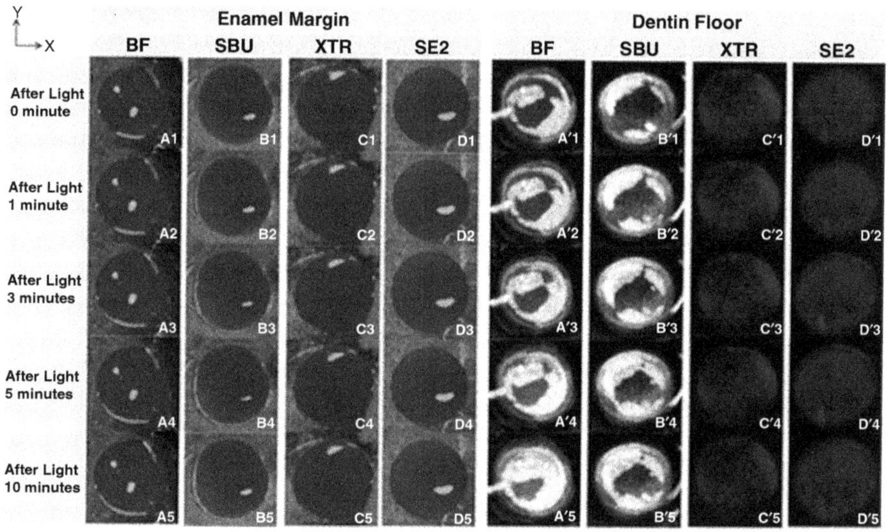

Fig. 3.2 Maximum intensity projection images from optical coherence tomography (OCT) three-dimensional (3D) data after light curing (**a–d, a′–d′**) at each time. At the enamel margins, Bond Force (seventh gen, BF), Scotchbond Universal Adhesive (universal, SBU), and OptiBond XTR (sixth gen, XTR) showed high signal intensity that progressed along the enamel interface after 10 min (**a1–a5, b1–b5, c1–c5**). On the other hand, Clearfil SE Bond 2 (sixth gen, SE2) did not show a high signal intensity at the enamel interface during the observation (**d1–d5**). At the dentin floors, BF and SBU showed bright areas that expanded at the floor after light curing for 10 min (**a′1–a′5, b′1–b′5**). On the other hand, XTR and SE2 showed almost no gap at the cavity floor during the observation (**c′1–c′5, d′1–d′5**)

3.4 Curing and Polymerization of the Adhesive

Light curing is the process to initiate and accelerate the free radical based polymerization reaction of the adhesive. As technology advanced, so did the light source evolve along with it and today it is possible to find LED light sources that emit multiple wavelengths, usually within the visible blue light spectrum. There are several factors that play a role in the equation that attempts to yield a high conversion ratio, minimize temperature increase, high power output [15, 16], light density [17], and time required [18]. Generally, the higher the output and flow of photons from the source, the quicker the reaction would be. It is possible in theory to create a light source that is strong enough to minimize curing time. The challenges facing that would be a high sharp increase in temperature that could have adverse effects on the pulp in vital teeth. Degree of conversion is another concern when using high intensity light curing devices [17, 19] Physical properties of the polymer also affect the ability of light to penetrate the deeper portions of the restoration [20], this is a result of how light passes through a non-clear composite material, but also a result of the propagation of the reaction unevenly across the restoration.

To ensure a restoration margin that has been well adapted with adhesive resin, the composite must copolymerize well with the bond in the extensions of the preparation. In the traditional incremental approach, this was successfully achieved with shallow composite layers, ensuring for repeated and excessive light exposure for polymerizing reactions. However, the bulk-fill technique blocks light from reaching the deepest extensions of the preparation. In other words, in the traditional incremental placement of composite, there are several separate light curing steps with each small layer of composite places. This gradually allows for maturation of the bond to dentin, and increased polymerization performance of the adhesive layer, due to increased irradiance. Therefore, a notable difference between traditional incremental placement of composite and bulk fill is several separate light curing with each layer of composite versus one large layer. Lack of sufficient light irradiation may inhibit complete curing of the composite and copolymerization of composite with the bond. In measuring the difference in polymerization completion at various depths, it was found that across various types and shades of traditional composites, incomplete polymerization occurred at greater depths using the bulk-fill technique, while no significant difference in hardness was observed at various depths using the incremental method [21].

In deep preparations with single increment fillings, the intensity of light reaching the adhesive is reduced due to the distance from the occlusal surface to the deep area such as the proximal gingival margin. In these cases, bulk filling will be a challenge since with a partially polymerized adhesive, the amount of light reaching the interface of the thick layer of bulk-fill composite and adhesive could be insufficient to establish a good seal. This is the reason why some researchers have advocated for application of a composite coating or intermediate layer in these areas prior bulk placement of the subsequent layer, to allow for improved polymerization of the adhesive-composite complex [22, 23]. With the challenges of bonding to deep dentin due to increased tubules density, orientation, and water content, it does appear that the bulk-fill strategy in this dentin region may be challenging without an additional resin-coating technique. Optical coherence tomography (OCT) experiments showed that compared to other conventional flowable materials, Surefill SDR Flow (Dentsply Sirona, Milford, DE) did have lower polymerization stress; in fact when applied in a bulk 2-mm increment to restore a dentin cavity, it showed perfect adaptation to the walls and floor. In contrast, the regular flowable composite, showed formation of gaps at the 2-mm deep cavity with the same type of one-step self-etch adhesive as was used for the bulk fill composite. However, when applied in one increment a 4-mm deep setup, both SDR and regular flowable showed interfacial defects [24].

It has been shown that the pattern of shrinkage stress for light-cured materials is from the bottom up in direction from the floor of the cavity to the top surface, placing a stretch on the adhesive layer with the largest vectors of polymerization stress at the deepest area of the preparation [25]. This is a critical issue for light-cured bulk-fill resin composites, particularly given the possibility of insufficient irradiation of the adhesive prior to and after placement of the composite. As mentioned earlier, in order to reach the post-gel phase, a sufficient intensity of light need to irradiate the composite and penetrate throughout the material to ensure curing of the deeper areas to achieve the cross-linking of the composite, as well as copolymerization with the adhesive layer and overall development of mechanical properties. One strategy in development of bulk-fill composite was increasing the overall translucency of the material to enable better light penetration, distribution and internal reflections [26].

A newly developed bulk-fill system incorporates high irradiance LED light curing unit (3 s PowerCure, Ivocalt-Vivadent AG, Schaan, Liechtenstein). The light curing process in this system takes only 3 s of irradiance using the light curing unit with high output (3000 mW/cm^2). When the high intensity light delivery was compared to the regular LED curing (1200 mW/cm^2), it was apparent that at the initial stage of composite polymerization, the high intensity system resulted in copolymerization between the bulk-fill composite and the adhesive at the cavity floor interface, which resisted against separation during polymerization. Overall, this light curing strategy together with increased translucency of the composite and improved photinitiator chemistry contributed to the maintenance of the composite bond to the deepest areas in the preparation [27].

Additionally, insufficient solvent evaporation from simplified adhesives may contribute to overall lower polymerization performance and quality of the adhesive layer. Therefore, application of an additional hydrophobic resin as a coating (such as a bonding agent) seem beneficial for these adhesives [28]. It was shown that mechanical properties of the polymerized bonding agent of a two-step self-etch adhesive was superior to that of an all-in-one adhesive from the same manufacturer with a similar composition [29].

Depending on the size and geometry of the preparation, homogeneity of the adhesive thickness may be another issue with single step adhesives. While the adhesive may pool in the preparation corner and create thick bond layer (up to 100 μm), it may be too thin at other areas (<5 μm) increasing the risk of a weak bond layer due to formation of an oxygen inhibition layer through most of the adhesive thickness [23]. The oxygen-inhibited layer is always produced as a thin soft and sticky superficial layer when a bonding resin is polymerized via free-radical initiation in air. In case of a super thin adhesive, the majority of the thickness will be oxygen-inhibited [30].

3.5 Adhesion of Bulk-Fill Dual-Cure Composites

Ducal cure composite systems have a combination of chemical initiators and light initiators materials. The goal of having dual cure materials is having the advantages in using light curing systems of speed for initial set, while combining the advantage of chemical cure that can provide a higher degree of conversion (DC) in deeper portions of the composite [31]. The slower initial chemical polymerization reaction preceding light activation has other advantages for the dual-cure bulk-fill resin composite; it permits viscoelastic flow within the material and stress relaxation as copolymerization occurs between the resin composite and adhesive at the bottom of the cavity. In other words, under such situation, there is more time for the composite-adhesive bond to mature due to the slower setting reaction of the composite. The depth of cure in an efficient self-cure system is not a function of light irradiance; however, a lower degree of cross-linking (i.e., more linear polymer) has been reported for self-cured materials. Even though the final DC in the self-cured mode may not be necessarily lower than the dual-cured mode, additional light-curing would improve the polymer cross-linking. This final light curing step may also contribute to the completion of copolymerization of composite and adhesive.

However, a concern that needs to be taken into account is the compatibility between the adhesive and bulk-fill composite. While light cured adhesive and composite systems are considered generally compatible, dual-cured bulk-fill composite may not be compatible with certain adhesives, particularly the all-in-one adhesives that use an acidic functional monomer. An adverse acid-base reaction with the basic tertiary amine of the dual-cure composite can prevent polymerization of the dual-cured composite [32]. This is why some adhesive manufacturers recommend the use of a dual-cure activator that mixes with the adhesive to reduce these adverse reactions with amine-based dual-cure composites. For example, Scotchbond Universal Adhesive must be mixed with its dual-cure activator (3 M ESPE, St Paul, MN, USA) containing sodium p-toluenesulfinate and ethanol, when an amine-based resin composite is used [32].

In order to address the adhesive incompatibilities, amine-free low-viscosity dual-cured bulk-fill resin composites have been introduced (such as BulkEZ, Danville Materials, Carlsbad, CA, USA). This material contains a proprietary hydroperoxide oxidizing agent and a thiourea reducing agent as the catalyst redox system that allows polymerization reaction within 2 min after mixing. The comparison of gap formation at the cavity floor among the dual-cure and several light-cured bulk-fill composites confirmed the advantage of the dual-cure approach in terms of bonding to a deep preparation.

3.6 The Issue of a Too Strong Bond

When the bonding to the tooth structure is strong enough to resist an uncontrolled polymerization shrinkage stress and there is no debonding or stress relaxation (through viscoelastic flow of the composite), the shrinkage stress could result in cuspal deflection, reduced bond strength, or worse, crack formation, and propagation. Another important finding in OCT real-time imaging study was the development of postcuring enamel cracks along the enamel walls, which was explained by the residual stress in the bulk-filled composite according to the postgel concept [33]. It is therefore evident that for a bulk-fill strategy to work, besides a good bonding ability, polymerization shrinkage management of the composite must be considered for the success of the restoration.

If a strong bond to dentin is successfully achieved, protecting the tooth and the bonded restoration from harmful stresses is the next challenge to tackle. Bulk-fill composites are not zero-shrinkage composites; therefore, the application of a stress-absorbing layer such as a resin-coating with flowable composite [23] or continuous fiber-reinforced composite layer [34] prior to bulk filling is recommended. Since shrinkage is an intrinsic resin property, reducing resin volume by adding non-monomer components such as organic or non-organic fillers has been considered as an effective way to reduce the magnitude of shrinkage. Incorporation of plasma-treated leno-weaved ultra-high molecular-weight polyethylene fiber (Ribbond, Seattle, WA) at the base of a deep cavity carried such an effect on polymerization shrinkage, while enhancing physical properties of the composite and potentially acting as a crack stopping mechanism (Fig. 3.3).

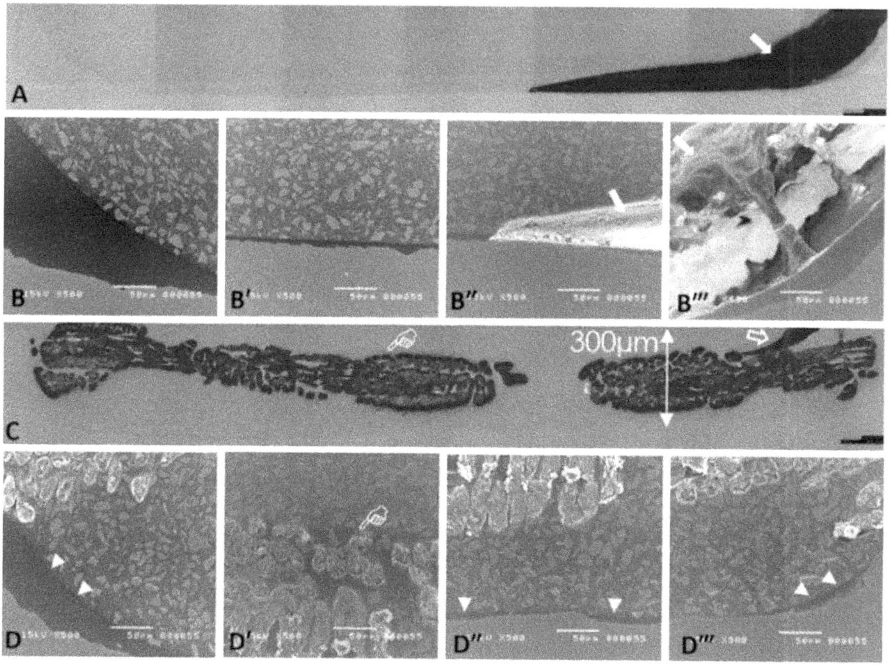

Fig. 3.3 Cross-sectional microscopic images of composite adaptation at 4-mm deep cavity bottom. (**a**) confocal laser scanning microscopy (CLSM) of the cavity floor in bulk-filled composite shows debonding of composite (Surefil) at the line angle. (**b**, **b**′, **b**″, and **b**‴) SEM images of the cross section in (**a**), it appears that polymerization shrinkage has pulled away the composite from the bonding layer (bold white arrow). (**c**) CLSM image of the cavity floor shows that fiber-reinforced increment reached a thickness of approximately 0.3 mm. A gap can be observed between the bulk placed composite and fiber-reinforced layer in **c** (blank arrow). (**d**, **d**′, **d**″, and **d**‴) SEM images of the cavity floor cross section presented in C, good adaptation of with fiber-reinforced increment at all interfaces can be observed (arrowheads)

3.7 Conclusion

Based on our current knowledge bonding of a bulk-fill composite to deep dentin is a possibility as long as the challenges of polymerization efficiency in depth and polymerization shrinkage stress have been addressed with the state-of-the-art technologies such as the enhanced light-cure or dual-cure mechanisms described in this chapter. Addition of continuous fiber would add value to stress distribution and protection of the bond to dentin. Clinicians are advised to select the most suitable bonding strategy for their bulk-fill technique, which appear to the authors of this chapter to be multi-step adhesives that have a separate hydrophobic bonding agent, namely the three-step etch-and-rinse (fourth gen) or the two-step self-etch (sixth gen) adhesive.

References

1. Van Meerbeek B, Yoshihara K, Van Landuyt K, Yoshida Y, Peumans M. From Buonocore's pioneering acid-etch technique to self-adhering restoratives. A status perspective of rapidly advancing dental adhesive technology. J Adhes Dent. 2020;22(1):7–34.
2. Sadr A, Nikaido T, Takagaki T, Hariri I, Nazari A, Tagami J. Ultra-morphological and nano-mechanical characterization of reinforced enamel and dentin by self-etch adhesives: the super tooth. J Nano Res. 2012;16:131–40.
3. Matsui N, Takagaki T, Sadr A, Ikeda M, Ichinose S, Nikaido T, et al. The role of MDP in a bonding resin of a two-step self-etching adhesive system. Dent Mater J. 2015;34(2):227–33.
4. Nazari A, Shimada Y, Sadr A, Tagami J. Pre-etching vs. grinding in promotion of adhesion to intact enamel using self-etch adhesives. Dent Mater J. 2012;31(3):394–400.
5. Turkistani A, Nakashima S, Shimada Y, Tagami J, Sadr A. Microgaps and demineralization progress around composite restorations. J Dent Res. 2015;94(8):1070–7.
6. Hu X, Luong MN, Zhang H, Zhu H, Chan DC, Sadr A. Influence of phosphoric acid etching on the dentin bond durability of universal adhesives. J Adhes Sci Technol. 2019;33(21):2356–68.
7. de Oliveira da Rosa WL, Piva E, da Silva AF. Bond strength of universal adhesives: a systematic review and meta-analysis. J Dent. 2015 Jul;43(7):765–76.
8. Tabata T, Shimada Y, Sadr A, Tagami J, Sumi Y. Assessment of enamel cracks at adhesive cavosurface margin using three-dimensional swept-source optical coherence tomography. J Dent. 2017;61:28–32.
9. Alshahni RZ, Shimada Y, Zhou Y, Yoshiyama M, Sadr A, Sumi Y, et al. Cavity adaptation of composite restorations prepared at crown and root: optical assessment using SS-OCT. Dent Mater J. 2019;38(5):779–89.
10. Klee JE, Renn C, Elsner O. Development of novel polymer technology for a new class of restorative dental materials. J Adhes Dent. 2020;22(1):35–45.
11. Versluis A, Tantbirojn D, Douglas WH. Do dental composites always shrink toward the light? J Dent Res. 1998;77(6):1435–45.
12. Sadr A, Ghasemi A, Shimada Y, Tagami J. Effects of storage time and temperature on the properties of two self-etching systems. J Dent. 2007;35(3):218–25.
13. Van Landuyt KL, Peumans M, De Munck J, Lambrechts P, Van Meerbeek B. Extension of a one-step self-etch adhesive into a multi-step adhesive. Dent Mater. 2006;22(6):533–44.
14. Hayashi J, Shimada Y, Tagami J, Sumi Y, Sadr A. Real-time imaging of gap progress during and after composite polymerization. J Dent Res. 2017;96(9):992–8.

15. Bouschlicher MR, Rueggeberg FA. Effect of ramped light intensity on polymerization force and conversion in a photoactivated composite. J Esthet Restor Dent. 2000;12(6):328–39.
16. Lovell LG, Newman SM, Donaldson MM, Bowman CN. The effect of light intensity on double bond conversion and flexural strength of a model, unfilled dental resin. Dent Mater. 2003;19(6):458–65.
17. Sakaguchi RL, Berge HX. Reduced light energy density decreases post-gel contraction while maintaining degree of conversion in composites. J Dent. 1998;26(8):695–700.
18. Lovell LG, Lu H, Elliott JE, Stansbury JW, Bowman CN. The effect of cure rate on the mechanical properties of dental resins. Dent Mater. 2001;17(6):504–11.
19. Silikas N, Eliades G, Watts DC. Light intensity effects on resin-composite degree of conversion and shrinkage strain. Dent Mater. 2000;16(4):292–6.
20. Emami N, Söderholm K-JM, Berglund LA. Effect of light power density variations on bulk curing properties of dental composites. J Dent. 2003;31(3):189–96.
21. Lazarchik DA, Hammond BD, Sikes CL, Looney SW, Rueggeberg FA. Hardness comparison of bulk-filled/transtooth and incremental-filled/occlusally irradiated composite resins. J Prosthet Dent. 2007;98(2):129–40.
22. Han S-H, Sadr A, Shimada Y, Tagami J, Park S-H. Internal adaptation of composite restorations with or without an intermediate layer: effect of polymerization shrinkage parameters of the layer material. J Dent. 2019;80:41–8.
23. Yahagi C, Takagaki T, Sadr A, Ikeda M, Nikaido T, Tagami J. Effect of lining with a flowable composite on internal adaptation of direct composite restorations using all-in-one adhesive systems. Dent Mater J. 2012;31(3):481–8.
24. Nazari A, Sadr A, Shimada Y, Tagami J, Sumi Y. 3D assessment of void and gap formation in flowable resin composites using optical coherence tomography. J Adhes Dent. 2013;15(3):237–43.
25. Cho E, Sadr A, Inai N, Tagami J. Evaluation of resin composite polymerization by three dimensional micro-CT imaging and nanoindentation. Dent Mater. 2011;27(11):1070–8.
26. Ferracane JL. Placing dental composites—a stressful experience. Oper Dent. 2008;33(3): 247–57.
27. Hayashi J, Tagami J, Chan D, Sadr A. New bulk-fill composite system with high irradiance light polymerization: integrity and degree of conversion. Dent Mater. 2020;36(12):1615–23.
28. Sadr A, Shimada Y, Tagami J. Effects of solvent drying time on micro-shear bond strength and mechanical properties of two self-etching adhesive systems. Dent Mater. 2007;23(9):1114–9.
29. Sadr A, Shimada Y, Lu H, Tagami J. The viscoelastic behavior of dental adhesives: a nanoindentation study. Dent Mater. 2009;25(1):13–9.
30. Yamaji A, Koga K, Tsujimoto A, Shimizu Y, Tsubota K, Takamizawa T, et al. Influence of oxygen-inhibited layer on dentin bond strength of chemical-cured resin composite. Eur J Oral Sci. 2013;121(5):497–503.
31. Feilzer AJ, de Gee AJ, Davidson CL. Setting stresses in composites for two different curing modes. Dent Mater. 1993;9(1):2–5.
32. Meda EM, Rached RN, Ignácio SA, Fornazari IA, Souza EM. Effect of different adhesive strategies and time on microtensile bond strength of a CAD/CAM composite to dentin. Oper Dent. 2019;44(3):262–72.
33. Versluis A, Tantbirojn D, Douglas WH. Distribution of transient properties during polymerization of a light-initiated restorative composite. Dent Mater. 2004;20(6):543–53.
34. Sadr A, Bakhtiari B, Hayashi J, Luong MN, Chen Y-W, Chyz G, et al. Effects of fiber reinforcement on adaptation and bond strength of a bulk-fill composite in deep preparations. Dent Mater. 2020;36(4):527–34.

4 What Happens When I Irradiate a BFC?

David C. Watts and Hamad Algamaiah

A basic question is: *What is light?* Over the past three centuries, *particle* and *wave* models have competed for dominance. However, thanks to quantum theory, a truce has been declared. Paradoxically, both models are now considered to be "true." Light behaves as a stream of particles (*photons*), but collectively—or even single photons—exhibit wavelike character, including interference and diffraction. The photon (particle) concept is essential to explain the photoelectric effect, the mechanism behind the operation of digital cameras and solar roof panels.

In terms of waves, a light beam has a *wavelength* (λ): the distance between successive peaks or troughs. This can be re-expressed as a *frequency* (ν), reciprocally related via a simple equation involving the *velocity* (c) of light.

$$c = \nu \cdot \lambda \tag{4.1}$$

A beam of visible (white) light consists of a range (or *spectrum*) of wavelengths (or frequencies). As Isaac Newton showed, white light can be split via a glass prism into its constituent wavelength ranges, *from red to violet*, often denoted by the capital letters: ROYGBIV. As, James Clark Maxwell showed, theoretically, and Heinrich Hertz showed experimentally, visible light is merely a central part of the whole electromagnetic spectrum (Fig. 4.1) with *ultra-violet* (UV) extending beyond the violet and *infra-red* (IR) and radio waves extending beyond the red [1, 2].

According to the quantum theory, each photon of light has an energy (E) given by the product of its frequency (ν) and Max Planck's constant (h).

D. C. Watts (✉)
School of Medical Sciences and Photon Science Institute, University of Manchester, Manchester, UK
e-mail: david.watts@manchester.ac.uk

H. Algamaiah
Department of Restorative Dental Science, College of Dentistry, King Saud University, Riyadh, Saudi Arabia
e-mail: haljamaiah@KSU.edu.sa

J. Sabbagh, R. McConnell (eds.), *Bulk Fill Resin Composites in Dentistry*,
https://doi.org/10.1007/978-3-031-16388-3_4

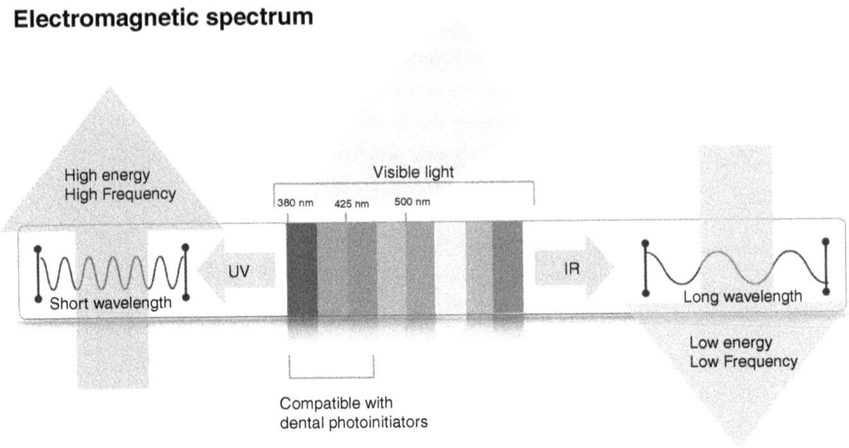

Fig. 4.1 Light of wavelengths visible to human eyes is a central part of the electromagnetic spectrum

$$E = h \cdot \nu = h \cdot c / \lambda \tag{4.2}$$

Planck's constant is almost unimaginably small (6.62607004 × 10^{-34} m^2 kg/s). Therefore, contrary to popular parlance, a *quantum leap* is the *smallest* possible change in energy! This also means that a solitary blue photon has only a small quantity of energy.

When using a light-curing unit (LCU), based around a light-emitting diode (LED) chip, the *Radiant Exitance* (mW/cm^2) is a measure of output ***power*** (Watts) *per unit area*. Power (W) is ***energy*** (Joules) *per unit time*. When we consider the light energy falling on a target surface, we use the term *Irradiance* (*I*), with the same units as radiant exitance. Thus, assuming irradiance remains constant, over time (*t*), the **radiant exposure** or energy (*E*) delivered is:

$$\text{Energy}\left(\text{J}/\text{cm}^2\right) = \text{Irradiance}\left(\text{W}/\text{cm}^2\right) \times \text{Time}\left(\text{s}\right)$$

or

$$E = I \cdot t \tag{4.3}$$

The above three equations are the main ones for understanding this subject. But understanding involves thinking about their physical meaning, magnitudes, and units, plus how they connect together.

When you use a torch or a light-curing unit, it is conceptually helpful to think of this as pumping out (irradiating) a continuous stream of photons. Even LCUs that deliver a relatively modest irradiance, are pumping out some *billion billion* (10^{18}) photons every second. However, these photons are not all necessarily "suitable". The criteria for suitability depends upon their frequency or spectral wavelength. Most LED-LCUs output visible blue light of wavelength circa 470 nm. But violet light chips may also be used, emitting at shorter wavelengths, circa 410 nm.

We must next consider *what happens to these photons?* There are two main questions:

1. How deeply do these photons penetrate into bulk fill RBCs?
2. What happens when a suitable photon meets a photo-sensitive molecule within the resin part of the resin-composite.

Before addressing these questions, let us briefly review the composition of RBCs that also applies to bulk fill formulations.

4.1 Formulation of RBCs

All RBCs are formulated with monomer (resin) mixtures that can be chemically *polymerized* to form a solid organic resin matrix. The near-universal types of monomer in current formulations are predominantly *dimethacrylates* that incorporate pairs of carbon–carbon double bonds (C=C) at either end of each monomer molecule. There are different types of organic structures between that vary in stiffness/flexibility and length (or size). It is the C=C bonds that undergo polymerization to create single C-C bonds in their place, linking the original monomers into linear or branched polymer networks, like beads on a necklace.

Pre-dispersed within the monomers are high volume-fractions of inorganic filler particles [3, 4]. These (mainly inert) particles are normally coated with a silane coupling agent that can co-polymerize with the resin matrix [5, 6]. These components are designed to create strong, stiff restorative materials that bear some comparison, both structurally and in properties, with the major tissues (enamel and particularly dentine) that the RBC is intended to repair. This outcome depends upon successful photopolymerization of the resin-phase. To achieve this goal, photo-initiator (PI) system molecules are also pre-dispersed within the resin-phase at a concentration of circa 1%.

4.1.1 Q1. Photon Penetration into RBCs

Firstly, before the stream of photons from the LCU optic tip reach the surface of the target composite, some may be lost if the optic tip is any distance from the target. This is due to the divergence angle of the light beam, whereby the irradiance generally decreases with distance from the tip [7–11]. That is why the distinction between *radiant emittance* and *irradiance* is important. These quantities are only numerically equal when the tip is in immediate proximity to the target. However, clinically, this is not always possible; for example, in a Class I or Class II cavity, the remaining cusps may create a "standoff" for the optic tip, above the occlusal surface of the restoration (Fig. 4.2).

Secondly, when light is incident on the RBC-paste surface a significant fraction may be *reflected* back, as expressed by the quantity **r** in Eq. (4.4).

Thirdly, the light that penetrates into the top surface of the composite may be subject to *attenuation* via two main processes: (1) absorption and (2) scattering. The

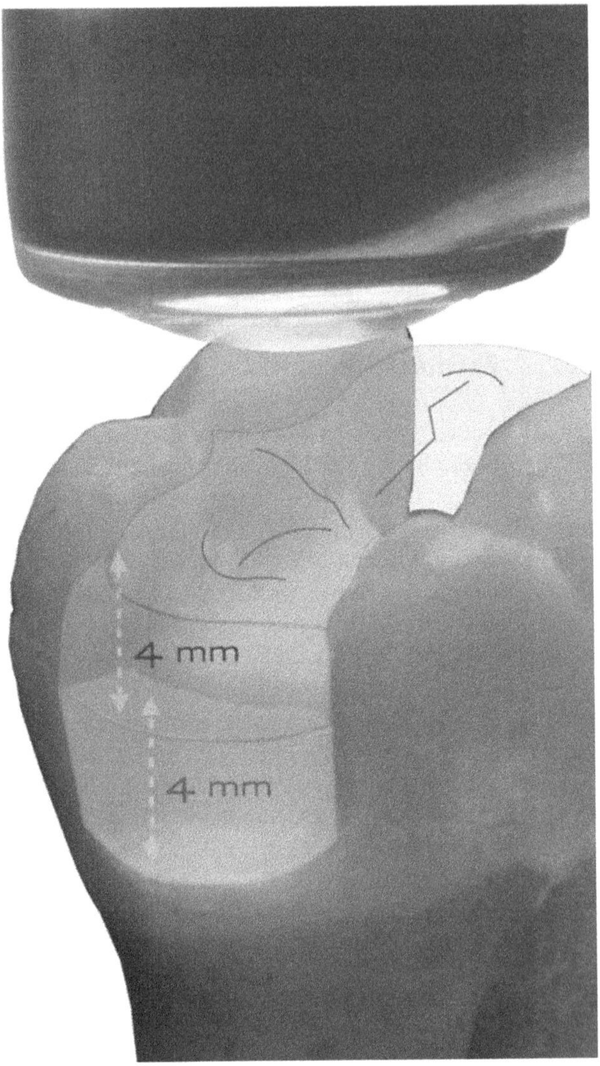

Fig. 4.2 Even with direct contact of the light guide tip and the occlusal surface, there can be a finite distance to the proximal box

combined effect of these processes is characterized by the Beer–Lambert law [12] that expresses an exponential *decrease* of irradiance (***I***) with depth (**d**), with an *attenuation coefficient* (μ).

$$I = I_0 (1 - r) \cdot e^{-\mu \cdot d} \tag{4.4}$$

where I_0 is the irradiance incident upon the top surface and **r** is the fraction of light undergoing specular reflection from the surface.

$$\mu = \mu_a + \mu_s \tag{4.5}$$

The attenuation coefficient is the sum of the coefficients for absorption and scattering, as per Eq. (4.5),

Scattering of light is commonplace at internal interfaces, especially where there is a change of *refractive index* (n) between two phases, such as resin and filler particles [13]. Some bulk fill RBCs incorporated quantities of short fibres. These are normally arranged in random orientations: their spatial distribution being *isotropic* (equal in all directions). Consequently, they exhibit no special optical phenomena. Scattering increases appreciably with shorter wavelengths, so blue light penetrates more than violet light [14, 15]. Filler-particle size (or fibre diameter) has a major effect [13, 16, 17]. Often particle or fibre diameters are *greater* than the wavelength of light (ca. 470 nm or 0.47 μm), so the light beam "sees" the particles and is refracted as it passes through, i.e. scattered from its original direction of travel [16, 17]. By contrast, nanoparticles (ca. 100 nm) are not "seen" by the light beam and so do not scatter light. The art and science of RBC formulation takes these physical factors into account to mitigate undesired effects. This has been particularly critical in designing bulk fill materials with optimized light transmission and using high efficiency photo-initiator mixtures.

Absorption of light occurs as photons encounter: (a) pigment molecules or similar species and (b) photo-initiator molecules. We will now consider PI systems in more detail.

4.1.2 Q2. Photons Encounter PI Molecules

Photo-sensitive compounds occur rather widely in the natural world. The best known is *chlorophyll* in plants and cyanobacteria; its green colour is due to the fact that it mainly absorbs blue and red wavelengths from sunlight.

Within dental RBCs, *suitable* photo-initiator systems respond to (absorb) visible blue and/or violet light (Fig. 4.3). This starts a photochemical process that initiates *free-radical addition polymerization* reactions. PI systems may be classified into two types: Norrish Type I and Norrish Type II. Camphorquinone/amine was the first

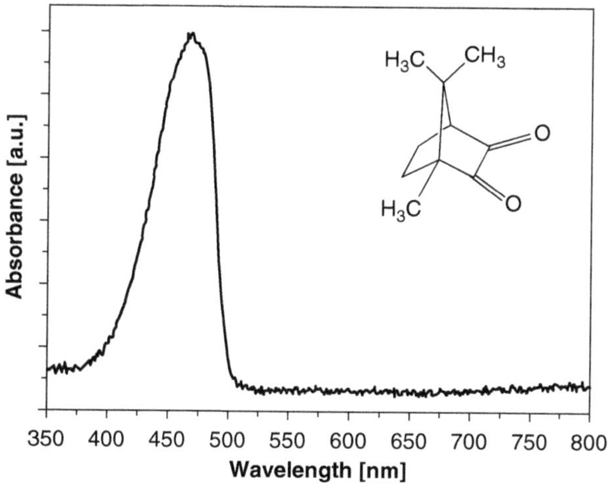

Fig. 4.3 The photo-initiator camphoroquinone absorbs light in the blue region of the visible spectrum

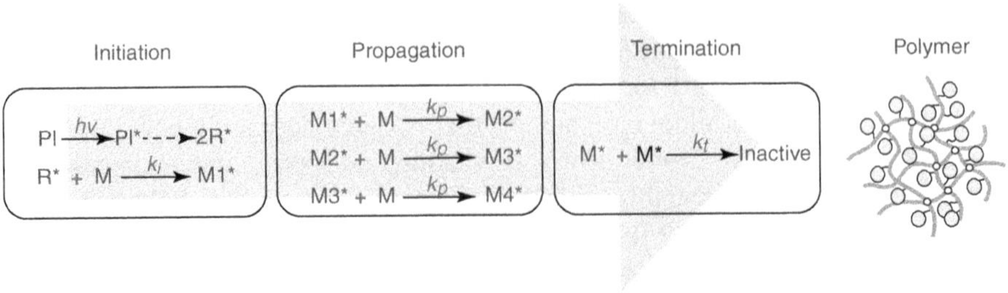

Fig. 4.4 Free-radical polymerization involves successive steps. *Initiation* creates monomer molecules with unpaired electrons. During *propagation* these radicals combine with further monomers forming growing polymer chains. Eventually the growth process stops due to one or more *termination* reactions

system to be developed for dental RBCs and this is Type II. More recently, Type I systems have also been used that involve a simpler bond-cleavage mechanism. Both types result in the formation of free radicals; i.e. highly reactive molecules with an unpaired electron. The propagation of the polymerization reaction involves radical-ended chains reacting with successive monomer molecules (Fig. 4.4).

Suitability, of a PI system, means that it corresponds to or matches the output wavelengths of the light-curing unit, by having an absorption band within the output wavelength range [18, 19]. Comparison might be made with a successful postal delivery. It is not sufficient to take a letter or parcel to a destination; there must be a letter box large enough to receive the letter (unless the door is opened)! Therefore, the critical light energy "*delivered*" is that which actually reaches its intended destination *and is absorbed* [20–22].

The types of monomer used to form dental resin matrices are mainly dimethacrylates, such as bis-GMA and TEGDMA. Each monomer has two methacrylate groups; one at either end. These are commonly represented by their principal feature: C=C. That is, a carbon–carbon *double* bond. In consequence, polymerization results in extensive cross-linking which creates a 3D network structure, rather than either linear or branched polymer chains [23]. Formation of this network structure causes a rapid increase in *elastic modulus* (i.e., stiffness, per unit cross-section) and an increase in local molecular density [23, 24], that corresponds to bulk polymerization shrinkage [25, 26].

It should be clearly understood that the irradiation, or photon dose "delivery", functions as a "trigger" such that the reaction continues long after the light has been switched OFF. However, the reaction continues only in regions of the material initially reached by photons and thus where free radicals have been generated. The initial phase of the reaction kinetics is marked by an auto-acceleration until a point is quickly reached when auto-deceleration sets in and further progress occurs increasingly slowly [27]. By this point the material is transitioning into the glassy state and internal movement of residual free radicals is slow [23, 24].

Once the composite has reached a hard glassy consistency, slow continued polymerization of the resin-phase is manifest by an increase in surface and bulk properties. Thus, surface hardness is known to gradually increase over periods of 1 month, or longer. However, intra-orally, water sorption may serve to soften surface layers [28].

4.2 Degree of Conversion

The kinetics (speed) of the polymerization process can be followed in a science lab by several complementary techniques. These include infra-red spectroscopy and monitoring shrinkage changes of the RBC that generally keep in step with the underlying polymerization reactions.

The most widely referenced quantity for expressing the immediate molecular "success" of photopolymerization is the Degree of Conversion (**DC**). **DC** of a composite surface or thin film is the percentage of C=C *double* bonds within the monomer molecules that have "disappeared" or rather converted to C-C single-bonds by polymerization. **DC** is measurable by infra-red spectroscopy [29, 30]. For a well-polymerized dimethacrylate composite **DC** is typically in the range 60–70%, not at all close to 100% (Fig. 4.5).

The reason for **DC**% values much less than 100% is that polymerization of these cross-linking molecules is a self-limiting process. As the monomer begins to polymerize, viscosity rises rapidly and within seconds the material has vitrified (entered the glassy state of matter), so the network becomes topologically entangled and the mobility that is requisite for further reaction is either greatly reduced or becomes impossible.

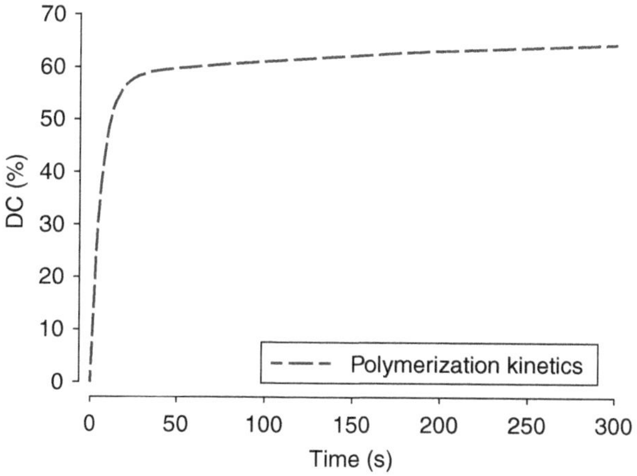

Fig. 4.5 During dimethacrylate photopolymerization, as shown over a linear timescale, the *degree of conversion* normal increases rapidly and then—more slowly—approaches a maximum value: ca. 60%. Complete 100% conversion is not reached at oral temperatures because formation of the cross-linked network is increasingly a self-limiting process as the material converts from a mobile paste to a hard solid

DC is the main parameter used to express the state of the polymer network in RBCs. However, even starting with the same monomers *different network structures* may be generated that nevertheless have the *same* **DC**. This will be the case if the different structures exhibit variations in their cross-link densities. Such an outcome can arise by using ultra-rapid curing versus slower photo-curing. Solvent swelling measurements can give an indication of such differences. More exact characterization involves X-ray diffraction experiments using synchrotron light sources.

4.3 "Bleaching" of Photo-Initiators and Colour Stability of BF-RBCs

Widely used Type II photo-initiators, such as camphorquinone (CQ), are yellowish compounds precisely because they absorb blue wavelengths from white light. When CQ molecules react photochemically they are "destroyed" and so lose their yellow appearance. This is termed "bleaching" of the PI. Ideally the amount of CQ formulated is just sufficient for the photochemical reaction, leaving no residual CQ. Otherwise the RBC may have an undesired yellow appearance. Additionally, CQ is used with an amine molecule (co-initiator). Again, residual amines can change chemically and develop a yellow appearance over time, thereby affecting the colour stability of the RBC. Managing this situation by the clinician is mainly down to: (a) being aware of the potential problem and (b) selecting RBC products that are known to be less susceptible to this problem.

4.4 The Reciprocity Hypothesis

As noted in Eq. (4.3), above, the light energy applied to the material is, by definition, the product of **irradiance** (***I***) and irradiation **time** (***t***). The first photo-cured dental resin-composites were considered to require irradiation for $t = 60$ s. Subsequent developments have enabled irradiation times to be reduced from 60 > 40 > 20 > 10 s, or—with specially formulated RBCs—even shorter times: >5 > 3 s.

To some extent, there has been an implicit assumption of a *general reciprocity hypothesis* that: "the same photo-cure outcomes will result from applying essentially constant energy densities despite reciprocal variations in the irradiance and time-period" [31–36]. An assumption is thereby made that the *if the irradiance is increased sufficiently* the irradiation period may be *reduced proportionately* without incurring inadequate consequences. As a general rule, this reciprocity assumption is over-optimistic and could be seriously misleading. Resin-composites are not all created equal. Some have been specially formulated with advanced photo-initiator systems to permit ultra-rapid cure within 5 or even 3 s [34, 37]. In other cases, it has been proposed that there is theoretical and experimental support for reciprocity to apply to monomer systems incorporating Type I photo-initiators [32] or to composites possessing a certain range of viscosity [35]. But in other cases, there may be anomalies [33] or reciprocity only to a limited extent [36].

On this point some conclusions may be drawn:

- For some specially formulated RBCs and with matched LCUs, ultra-rapid cure may be safe and feasible.
- With the majority of composites on the market, it is best not to assume exact reciprocity but to apply a safety factor of at least 2, especially with darker composite shades. That means irradiating for *at least double* the time corresponding to exact reciprocity. And even then, a means of checking the radiant emittance of the LCU is essential.

4.5 Shrinkage Phenomena

During polymerization of dimethacrylate monomers, the conversion of C=C bonds involves an *intrinsic densification* or shrinkage as the original *inter*-molecular spacings between individual monomer molecules are replaced by shorter C-C bonds creating the polymeric chains. As the proportion of the resin-monomer phase is reduced by addition of filler particles so the overall shrinkage is reduced. Nevertheless, even the most optimal RBC formulations exhibit some shrinkage. Shrinkage by itself is not the problem, but shrinkage stress—that arises when the RBC is photo-cured in the confined space of a cavity. When non-bulk fill composites are placed in a deep cavity, the traditional means of mitigating stress is to place the material incrementally. Bulk fill composites are intended to obviate the necessity for incremental placement. The good news is that, with many recent formulations, shrinkage phenomena are moderate [38]. Manufacturers have striven to design and formulate against excessive shrinkage. Since RBC placement is both an art and a science the practitioner can resolve to learn more about optimal placement with different cavity shapes, sizes and designs.

4.6 Photo-Curing of Highly Filled Systems Following Pre-Heating or Sonication

There are several highly filled composite systems available that require either pre-heating [39] or sonication before bulk placement. The effect of these pre-treatments is to enhance flowability and thus reduce the viscosity to ensure good cavity adaptation. Once placed in the cavity these materials revert to a stiff and carveable consistency. When the desired occlusal anatomy has been achieved it is vital to proceed to apply the recommended photo-cure procedures. Without that essential step, clinical failure is certain!

4.7 Depth of Cure

Finally, since we are considering bulk fill composites, we consider *Depth of Cure* (**DoC**).

Bulk fill composites are, by definition, those having a **DoC** of 4 mm or greater. The practitioner should note specific manufacturer claims for each product. These should include the precise irradiation regime that should be followed. Further details of how Depth of Cure can be verified and validated are presented in the following Chap. 5.

References

1. Maxwell JC. VIII. A dynamical theory of the electromagnetic field. Philos Trans R Soc Lond A. 1865;155:459–512.
2. Maxwell JC. The scientific papers of James clerk Maxwell. Cambridge: Cambridge University Press; 1890.
3. Bowen R. Properties of a silica-reinforced polymer for dental restorations. J Am Dent Assoc. 1963;66(1):57–64.
4. Cramer N, Stansbury J, Bowman C. Recent advances and developments in composite dental restorative materials. J Dent Res. 2011;90(4):402–16.
5. Lung CYK, Matinlinna JP. Aspects of silane coupling agents and surface conditioning in dentistry: an overview. Dent Mater. 2012;28(5):467–77.
6. Chen M-H. Update on dental nanocomposites. J Dent Res. 2010;89(6):549–60.
7. Caldas D, Almeida J, Correr-Sobrinho L, Sinhoreti M, Consani S. Influence of curing tip distance on resin composite Knoop hardness number, using three different light curing units. Oper Dent. 2003;28(3):315–20.
8. Price RB, Derand T, Sedarous M, Andreou P, Loney RW. Effect of distance on the power density from two light guides. J Esthet Restor Dent. 2000;12(6):320–7.
9. Corciolani G, Vichi A, Davidson CL, Ferrari M. The influence of tip geometry and distance on light-curing efficacy. Oper Dent. 2008;33(3):325–31.
10. Ilie N, Watts DC. Outcomes of ultra-fast (3 s) photo-cure in a RAFT-modified resin-composite. Dent Mater. 2020;36:570–9.
11. Thomé T, Steagall W Jr, Tachibana A, Braga RM, Turbino ML. Influence of the distance of the curing light source and composite shade on hardness of two composites. J Appl Oral Sci. 2007;15(6):486–91.
12. Swinehart DF. The Beer-Lambert law. J Chem Educ. 1962;39(7):333.
13. Shortall A, Palin W, Burtscher P. Refractive index mismatch and monomer reactivity influence composite curing depth. J Dent Res. 2008;87(1):84–8.
14. Shimokawa C, Sullivan B, Turbino M, Soares C, Price RB. Influence of emission spectrum and irradiance on light curing of resin-based composites. Oper Dent. 2017;42(5):537–47.
15. Harlow J, Rueggeberg F, Labrie D, Sullivan B, Price RB. Transmission of violet and blue light through conventional (layered) and bulk cured resin-based composites. J Dent. 2016;53:44–50.
16. Fronza B, Ayres A, Pacheco R, Rueggeberg F, Dias C, Giannini M. Characterization of inorganic filler content, mechanical properties, and light transmission of bulk-fill resin composites. Oper Dent. 2017;42(4):445–55.
17. Emami N, Sjödahl M, Söderholm K-JM. How filler properties, filler fraction, sample thickness and light source affect light attenuation in particulate filled resin composites. Dent Mater. 2005;21(8):721–30.

18. Rueggeberg FA, Giannini M, Arrais CAG, Price RBT. Light curing in dentistry and clinical implications: a literature review. Braz Oral Res. 2017;31(suppl 1):e61. https://doi.org/10.1590/1807-3107BOR-2017.vol31.0061.
19. Rueggeberg FA. State-of-the-art: dental photocuring—a review. Dent Mater. 2011;27(1):39–52.
20. Price R, Ferracane J, Shortall A. Light-curing units: a review of what we need to know. J Dent Res. 2015;94(9):1179–86.
21. Mutluay MM, Rueggeberg FA, Price RB. Effect of using proper light-curing techniques on energy delivered to a class 1 restoration. Quintessence Int. 2014;45(7):549–56.
22. Price RB, McLeod ME, Felix CM. Quantifying light energy delivered to a class I restoration. J Can Dent Assoc. 2010;76(2):a23.
23. Stansbury JW, Dickens SH. Network formation and compositional drift during photo-initiated copolymerization of dimethacrylate monomers. Polymer. 2001;42(15):6363–9.
24. Dickens SH, Stansbury J, Choi K, Floyd C. Photopolymerization kinetics of methacrylate dental resins. Macromolecules. 2003;36(16):6043–53.
25. Watts D, Marouf A, Al-Hindi A. Photo-polymerization shrinkage-stress kinetics in resin-composites: methods development. Dent Mater. 2003;19(1):1–11.
26. Algamaiah H, Sampaio CS, Rigo LC, Janal MN, Giannini M, Bonfante EA, et al. Microcomputed tomography evaluation of volumetric shrinkage of bulk-fill composites in class II cavities. J Esthet Restor Dent. 2017;29(2):118–27.
27. Burtscher P. Stability of radicals in cured composite materials. Dent Mater. 1993;9(4):218–21.
28. Watts DC, Amer O, Combe EC. Surface hardness development in light-cured composites. Dent Mater. 1987;3(5):265–9.
29. Imazato S, McCabe JF, Tarumi H, Ehara A, Ebisu S. Degree of conversion of composites measured by DTA and FTIR. Dent Mater. 2001;17(2):178–83.
30. Stansbury J, Dickens SH. Determination of double bond conversion in dental resins by near infrared spectroscopy. Dent Mater. 2001;17(1):71–9.
31. Musanje L, Darvell BW. Polymerization of resin composite restorative materials: exposure reciprocity. Dent Mater. 2003;19(6):531–41.
32. Wydra JW, Cramer NB, Stansbury JW, Bowman CN. The reciprocity law concerning light dose relationships applied to BisGMA/TEGDMA photopolymers: theoretical analysis and experimental characterization. Dent Mater. 2014;30(6):605–12.
33. Hadis M, Leprince J, Shortall A, Devaux J, Leloup G, Palin WM. High irradiance curing and anomalies of exposure reciprocity law in resin-based materials. J Dent. 2011;39(8):549–57.
34. Gorsche C, Griesser M, Gescheidt G, Moszner N, Liska R. β-Allyl sulfones as addition–fragmentation chain transfer reagents: a tool for adjusting thermal and mechanical properties of dimethacrylate networks. Macromolecules. 2014;47(21):7327–36.
35. Palagummi SV, Hong T, Wang Z, Moon CK, Chiang MY. Resin viscosity determines the condition for a valid exposure reciprocity law in dental composites. Dent Mater. 2020;36(2):310–9.
36. Sadeghyar A, Watts DC, Schedle A. Limited reciprocity in curing efficiency of bulk-fill resin-composites. Dent Mater. 2020;36:997–1008.
37. Algamaiah H, Silikas N, Watts DC. Conversion kinetics of rapid photo-polymerized resin composites. Dent Mater. 2020;36:1266–74.
38. Algamaiah H, Silikas N, Watts DC. Polymerization shrinkage and shrinkage stress development in ultra-rapid photo-polymerized bulk fill resin composites. Dent Mater. 2021;37:559–67.
39. Yang J, Silikas N, Watts DC. Pre-heating effects on extrusion force, stickiness and packability of resin-based composite. Dent Mater. 2019;35:1594–602.

How Do I Select and Deploy Light Curing Units for BFC?

5

Hamad Algamaiah and David C. Watts

5.1 What Are the Older LCU Technologies?

Firstly, we must identify older technologies that were acceptable and revolutionary when they were first introduced but are now superseded by superior technologies and designs.

Light curing units (LCUs) for dentistry normally must deliver light from the blue region of the visible spectrum that corresponds to the wavelength range over which photoinitiator(s) incorporated in resin-monomers can absorb energy. The first visible-light photoinitiator system for dentistry was developed and patented in 1975 at the Corporate Laboratories of *Imperial Chemical Industries* (ICI) PLC in the United Kingdom [1]. This used Camphoroquinone (CQ) as the photoabsorber in combination with an amine. CQ is a yellow compound, as it absorbs blue wavelengths (ca. 470 nm) from visible light.

The light-bulb technology used in the first LCUs, developed for dental use, is known as *Quartz Tungsten Halogen* (QTH). This consisted of an electrically heated tungsten wire enclosed in a quartz bulb containing a halogen gas. QTH bulbs emitted an *incandescent* white light (all visible wavelengths) plus infra-red radiation that resulted in considerable heat generation in the bulb and any surrounding material. QTH bulbs were formerly used extensively for domestic lighting and in movie projectors.

H. Algamaiah
Department of Restorative Dental Science, College of Dentistry, King Saud University, Riyadh, Saudi Arabia
e-mail: haljamaiah@KSU.edu.sa

D. C. Watts (✉)
School of Medical Sciences and Photon Science Institute, University of Manchester, Manchester, UK
e-mail: david.watts@manchester.ac.uk

J. Sabbagh, R. McConnell (eds.), *Bulk Fill Resin Composites in Dentistry*,
https://doi.org/10.1007/978-3-031-16388-3_5

Dental QTH-LCU devices deliver a wide range of wavelength between 370 and 2500 nm [2]. Such a wide range is beyond the required wavelengths and necessitated the use of optical filters to remove unwanted wavelengths (greater than 515 nm). A cooling fan was also required to cool the filters and minimize heat conduction to the optic delivery tip, otherwise termed the 'light guide'. QTH-LCU devices were mainly designed in the form of a hand-held 'gun' and were almost invariably powered via a mains electrical cable, occasionally via a transformer unit. These devices undoubtedly worked, although their ergonomics were poor, particularly as irradiation times were in the range 40–60 s. Moreover, bulb life was relatively short, around 100 h of use, due to the fast degradation of the light bulb.

A further type of LCU was developed: Plasma-Arc devices. These devices were very expensive. They had better ergonomics in terms of a 'pen'-like design, with a cable attached. For economic reasons their uptake was low except in some regions such as the USA. Plasma light is generated between electrodes at high voltages in a bulb containing a gaseous mixture of ionized molecules (e.g., xenon, argon). The radiant output extended over all visible wavelengths and was of high 'intensity' (radiant exitance). This did facilitate shorter irradiation periods.

5.2 Selection Principles

As with all clinical dental equipment there is a wide range on the market: available direct from manufacturers, via established resellers or for purchase online. In the case of *Light Curing Units* (*LCUs*) not only are there different technologies available but significant variations in design, ergonomics, build quality, performance, energy efficiency, safety, and cost. The selection principles can be determined by answering the questions below:

Why are Light Emitting Diode (LED) Light Curing Units now dominant?

LEDs are generically solid-state devices that emit visible radiation when an electrical potential (voltage) is supplied to suitable materials. This *electroluminescence* was discovered by accident early in the last century and the first LED results were published in 1907 [3]. LEDs were forgotten only to be rediscovered in the 1920s and again in the 1950s. The first viable LEDs were by-products of research into semiconductor lasers. During the past 60 years, LEDs have become devices in-their-own-right and today are versatile light sources, with extensive domestic and industrial applications. State-of-the-art LEDs are small, rugged, reliable, bright, and efficient [4].

The emitted light from the LEDs is generated by LED chips, which consist of small semi-conductor layers. Supplied electrical energy is converted into radiant light emittance (Fig. 5.1). A particular feature of LED chips is that their output wavelength range is a narrow band: i.e. of a single colour. Thus, the first technical applications of LEDs in the 1950s were as low-power red or green lights on calculators and other small electronic devices. However, emitting blue light proved to be a difficult task, which took three more decades to achieve. It required the development of techniques for the growth of high-quality crystals as well as the ability to

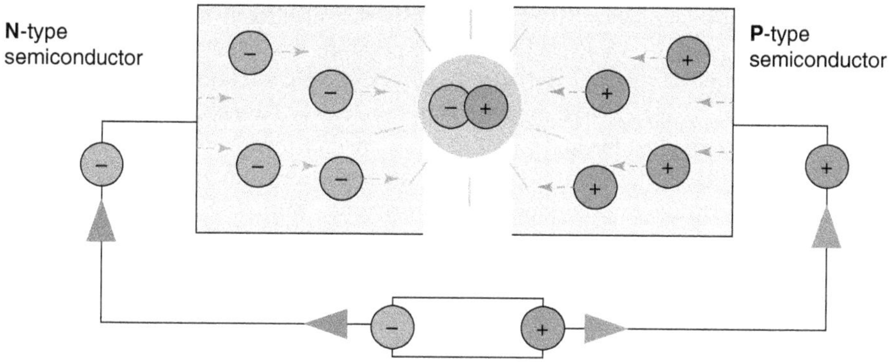

Fig. 5.1 How light is generated from a LED chip. The energy released (directly as a form of light) is caused by the combination of electrons (−) and holes (+) at the P-N junction

control p-doping of semiconductors with high bandgap, which was achieved with gallium-nitride (GaN) at the end of the 1980s. The development of efficient blue LEDs also required the production of GaN-based alloys with different compositions and their integration into multilayer structures. The 2014 Nobel Prize in Physics was awarded to three Japanese scientists for the invention of blue LEDs [5].

The development of blue-light LEDs was a great advance, which then enabled production of white LED devices—as used in domestic lighting, display screens, and the motor car industry. When exciting a phosphor material with a blue LED, light is emitted in the green and red spectral ranges, which, combined with the blue light, appears as white. Alternatively, multiple LEDs of complementary colours (red, green, and blue) can be used together.

The possible dental application of blue LEDs was first proposed by Mills in 1995 [6] and shown to be viable by Mills, Jandt, and Ashworth in 1999 [7]. At that time, the radiant emittance of LEDs was relatively low, so concentric arrays of LED chips were designed and patented [8] and the first dental LED-LCU publications appeared in 1999 [7, 9–12]. Production of commercial LED-LCU devices for dentistry really took off with the development of high irradiance single *LumiLed* chips [13].

Since a blue light source of sufficient radiant emittance was the pre-requisite for LCUs to excite CQ photoinitiator, it was inevitable that blue LEDs would be deployed for dentistry.

However, this coincided with a period where the original CQ/amine patent was expiring and when scientists were exploring variants and alternatives to the CQ type of photoinitiator (PI).

Photochemists classify PIs as Norrish type I and type II (See Chap. 4).

Some PIs absorb more strongly in the shorter-wavelength violet region (ca. 410 nm) as compared to the blue region (ca. 470 m). Combinations of PIs may be more efficient at promoting a higher degree-of-conversion (DC) of the resin monomers. Alternative PIs may also avoid any residual yellow coloration in the composite, post-irradiation. This is particularly important for design of white shades of resin composites for patients after tooth-whitening.

This situation of alternative photoinitiators has promoted the design and the commercial availability of LED-LCUs incorporating two types of LED chip—of either ca. 470 nm (blue) or ca. 410 nm (violet) peak-spectral output (Fig. 5.2) [14]. Some devices have one ca. 410 nm chip and three ca. 470 nm chips in a 2 × 2 array (Fig. 5.3). Accordingly, blue and violet photons are emitted together and emerge via the LCU-optic (light guide). Sometimes, such devices are named 'polywave' although that term may be commercially copyright. 'Multi-chip' is an acceptable alternative. Again, this type of output has been termed wideband or broadband. However, if these terms are used, it must be understood that the emitted spectrum consists of overlapping spectral peaks.

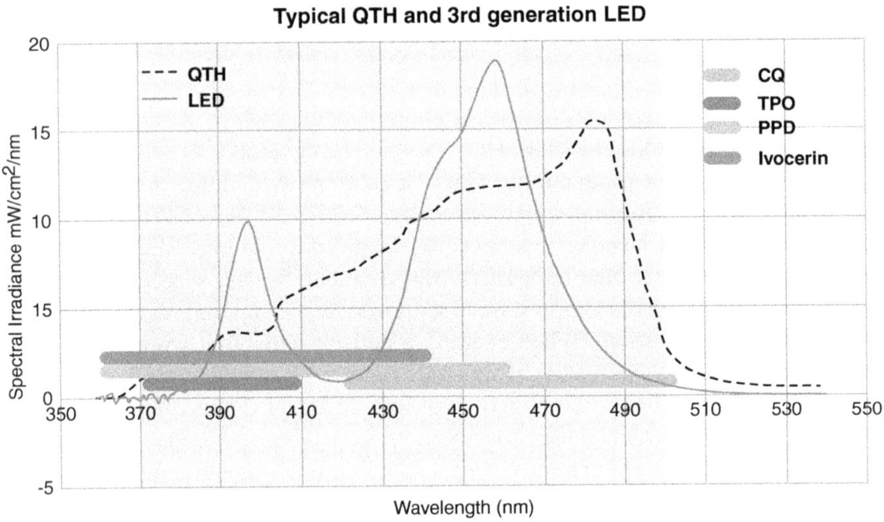

Fig. 5.2 Radiant exitance versus wavelength in the violet–blue region of the visible spectrum for (**a**) a filtered QTH light source (dashed line) and (**b**) a multi-chip LED source (solid line). The absorption bands for four types of photoinitiator molecule are also indicated

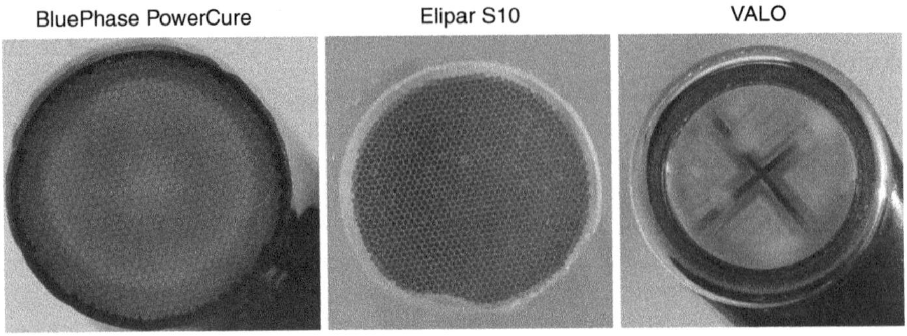

Fig. 5.3 Three examples of optic tips for LED-LCUs. The Bluephase and VALO lights have multi-chips, whereas the Elipar S10 has a single (blue) LED chip

Violet light—being of shorter wavelength than blue light—has reduced penetrative effectiveness through resin-based composites (RBCs), due to greater scattering and absorption effects. This may be significant when photo-curing bulk fill materials to 4 mm or greater depths.

What are the technical aspects and requirements for LED-LCUs?

As with most medical and dental devices there are appropriate regulations, such as the requirements for CE marking, that should be satisfied before marketing products. However, there are unregulated devices available for online purchase that may be hazardous in some circumstances. To understand these issues, we need to delve more deeply into regulatory requirements and technical performance details.

The *International Standards Organization* has produced a Standard (ISO 10650: 2018) for all LCU devices, which it refers to as *Powered Polymerization Activators* [15]. QTH devices are termed Class 1 and LED devices are termed Class 2. In both classes, Type 1 denotes 'powered with mains supply' and Type 2 denotes 'powered with rechargeable battery/capacitor'.

Are *Radiant Exitance* and *Irradiance* the same or different?

In everyday speech, the light delivered from any LCU is commonly referred to as its brightness or intensity. However, when the light output is quantified by a suitable *radiometric* instrument it is important to understand and use the correct technical terms and units.

In the International System of Units (SI), the *watt* (symbol: W) is a unit of *power* or radiant flux expressing the *rate* of *energy* transfer, equivalent to *joules per second*. As light emerges from the LCU light guide or 'optic' over a defined exit area, this is expressed as the *radiant exitance* (UNITS W/m^2 or mW/cm^2).

Light that *emerges* from a LCU light guide is then intended to fall on the 'target' material. When light falls—or is *incident*—on a surface, the amount of light *received* is termed the *Irradiance* (also mW/cm^2).

Based on the understanding of light as a stream of photons, the numerical value of irradiance is ultimately *proportional to* the *number of photons per second* over a given area. The actual photon number/sec is ca. 10^{18} or a billion-billion [16].

The *radiant exposure* is *the Irradiance* × *Time* of irradiation. It follows that this is *Energy* delivered per unit area: UNITS: $joules/cm^2$.

In the dental context, the LCU optic tip may be essentially in contact with the target material, placed, for example, in a Class V cavity. In such a situation, the Irradiance will be *numerically equal* to the radiant emittance. But in many situations, light travels some distance from the optic tip to reach the material. And over that distance the light beam may be divergent in cross-sectional area. Thus: *Irradiance may decrease with distance* from the optic tip (Fig. 5.4).

It is important that the clinician should:

- Know your materials and what the manufacturer recommends either by Radiant exposure or by Irradiance over a specific period of time;
- When purchasing a LED-LCU, if possible, find a graph that plots the Irradiance versus distance up to about 12 mm.

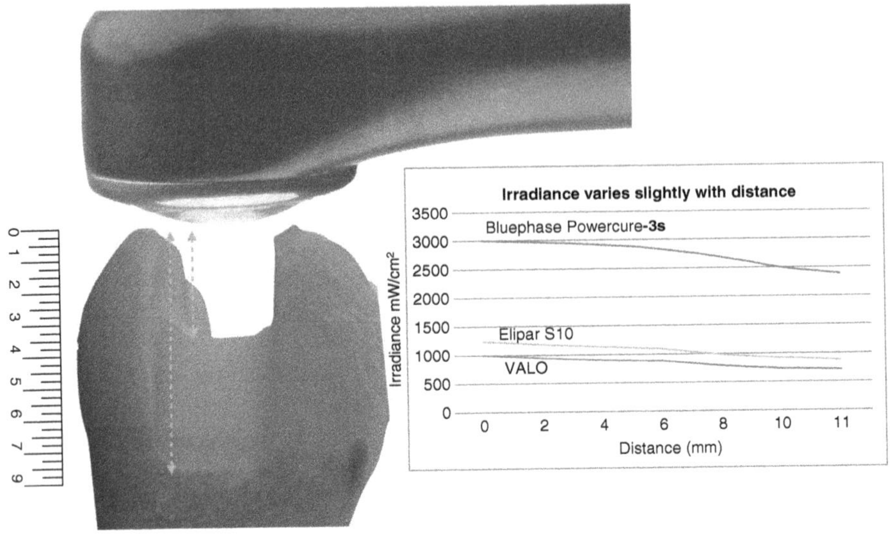

Fig. 5.4 Irradiance variations with distance (mm) from the optic tips of three LED-LCUs

For a LED-LCU device, is a 'wide-band' spectral output better than a 'narrow-band' output?

As already mentioned, light from LCUs is typically in the blue and/or violet region of the visible spectrum. When this light falls on a resin-based-composite only those photons that correspond to the absorption spectrum of the incorporated photoinitiator(s) will be absorbed (Figs. 5.2 and 5.3).

Manufacturers have been able to produce LED-LCU devices of increasing radiant exitance. This has led to concerns about excessive power that could be hazardous to both patient and operator. The current ISO Standard for Powered Polymerization Activators [15] thus has requirements that radiant exitance of devices *shall not exceed certain limits*, depending on the wavelength range, as follows:

380–515 nm range: The radiant exitance shall not be more than 40,000 W/m^2 (4000 mW/cm^2).

Below 380 nm (UV range): The radiant exitance shall be no more than 2000 W/m^2 (200 mW/cm^2).

Above 515 nm: The radiant exitance shall be no more than 1000 W/m^2 (100 mW/cm^2).

- Know your materials: use 'polywave' LCUs to irradiate any photoinitiator systems that require light from the violet spectrum.

What is a 'Beam Profile' and is it important?

When photons are emitted from the light guide of a LED-LCU it is tempting to assume that they are of *uniform and constant number density* across the surface of the optic tip. This cannot safely be assessed via direct visual assessment. And in any case, the human eye is not a radiometer as it does not respond equally to different wavelengths. Nevertheless, if the optic tip is covered by one or more sheets of paper, some indication of radiant variation might be perceived across the tip surface.

The ideal 'beam profile' may be likened to a top hat. However, many LED-LCUs vary by greater or lesser extents from such a profile, although those manufactured by reputable companies to not depart too drastically from the ideal. Moreover, some manufacturers have now achieved virtually 100% conformity to the 'top hat' ideal (Fig. 5.5). With time, the LCU's beam profile and efficiency may decrease due to tip deterioration, mostly due to autoclaving, disinfection sprays, or contamination by attached resin debris. Such resin debris could be in the centre of the beam hotspot which then could significantly reduce the irradiance. Thus, regular evaluation and maintenance is important.

It is concerning, however, that many inexpensive LED-LCUs marketed online have very poor beam profiles, exhibiting regions of low power (cold spots) and regions of dangerously excessive power (hot spots). As the measured radiant exitance is usually an average over the optic tip, an apparently acceptable average can be dangerously misleading.

- When purchasing a LED-LCU, request data (perhaps an image) of the beam profile, to confirm the homogeneity of the beam. This should have been determined by an appropriate method.

How do the ergonomics of LED-LCU devices vary?

Dental LED-LCU devices are designed in a variety of styles. Of these, 'pen' designs predominate over 'gun' designs. However, even then, there are considerable variations in the overall balance and feel. Some devices have an attached cable that plugs directly or indirectly into mains power.

Cable-free designs are widely available. The 'pen' incorporates a lithium-ion battery at the back of the pen and the 'light guide' at the front of the pen, with push-button controls and status displays on the upper surface of the pen, activated by the dentist's forefinger. The pen device can be charged by seating the back end into a compact base unit that may be sited conveniently at the chair-side.

Some devices are marketed with both cabled and cable-free options.

In most 'pen' designs there is no need for a fan to be incorporated. Silent operation is preferable for both patient and clinician.

A range of 'light guide tips' are generally available where these are interchangeable tips and can be removed for sterilization or covered by a plastic sleeve to avoid cross-contamination. Such tips may vary in exit-diameter and most are provided with a curve at the forward part of the light guide to permit direct occlusal irradiation. However, some alternate designs are without a detachable light guide, whereby light is emitted *perpendicularly* from the forward part of the LCU. These are generally smaller and lighter, permitting improved access to photo-cure molar restorations.

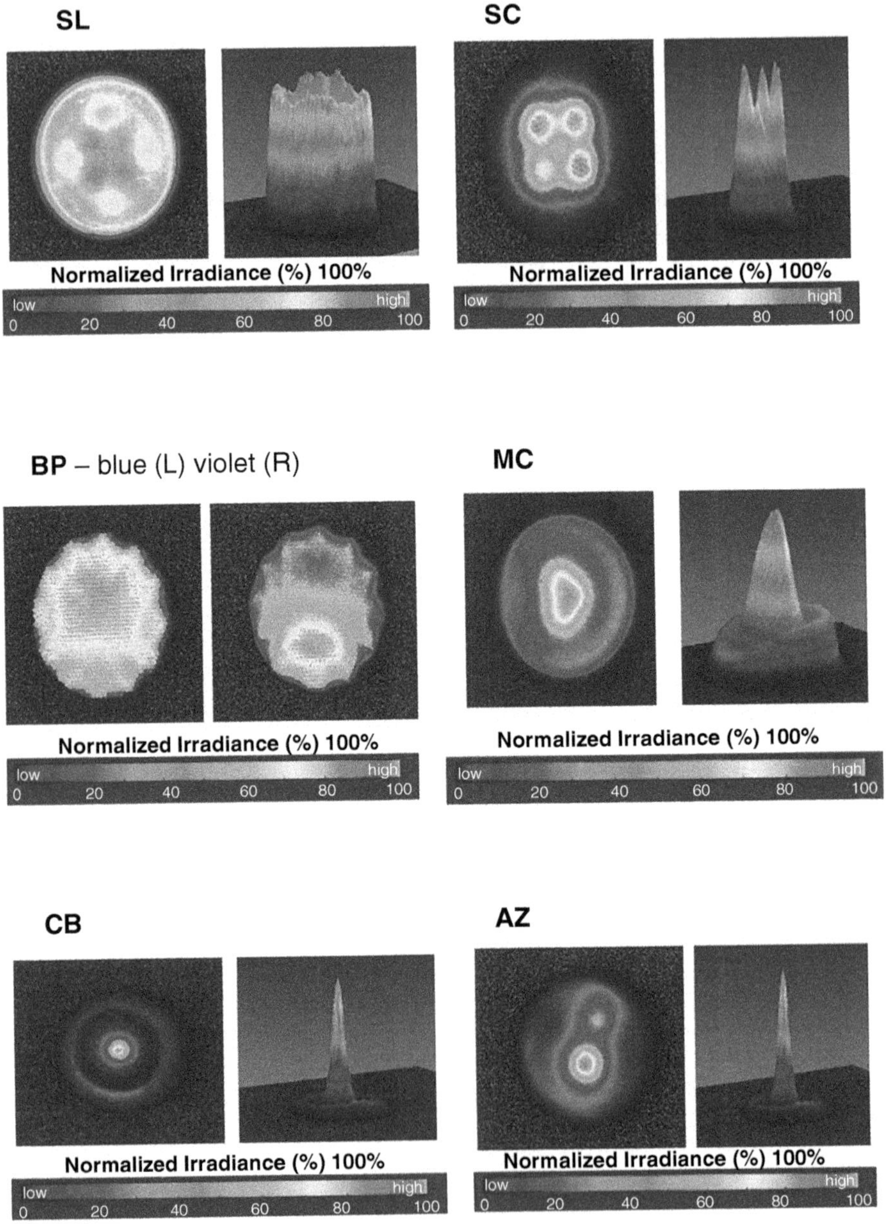

Fig. 5.5 Beam Profiles for six LED-LCUs, shown in 2D and 3D in each case, except for **BP**, where the blue and violet irradiance maps are presented. **SL** and **SC** exhibit essentially Top-Hat profiles. CB and AZ exhibit poor beam profiles, with distinct 'hot spots' and peripheral 'cold' regions

A notably sophisticated innovation, in a specific 'pen' design, is a feature assigned the registered name *PolyVision*™. This is particularly intended for use in conjunction with ultra-fast photocuring over a 3 s period [17]. It is analogous to 'lane assist' technology in a motor car, where an audible notification alerts a driver when they are straying out of their motorway (autobahn) lane. In a *Polyvision* LCU, a similar alert arises if the dentist moves their light guide tip away from their intended position over the restoration. It alerts the user of the improper operation by vibrating and automatically extends the exposure time by 10%, if necessary. If the movement may prevent the material from curing properly, the light will automatically interrupt the exposure cycle so that it can be repeated. This feature can itself be switched off, when desired.

- Based on your LED-LCU, make sure that the battery is always fully charged. Also, independent of the design, the light exiting the tip must be perpendicular to the restoration surface, covering the whole restoration surface area.

5.3 Before Deploying Light

5.3.1 Consider the Diameter of the LCU Tip

A range of different tip diameters are available. It is important to know the *active tip diameter* where this might affect the efficiency of polymerization (Fig. 5.6). For example, a curing tip might have a diameter of 10 mm^2, but an active tip diameter of only 8.5 mm^2. This might require a second curing cycle to cover the restorative surface. More importantly, if the beam profile is non-uniform, multiple curing positions may be necessary.

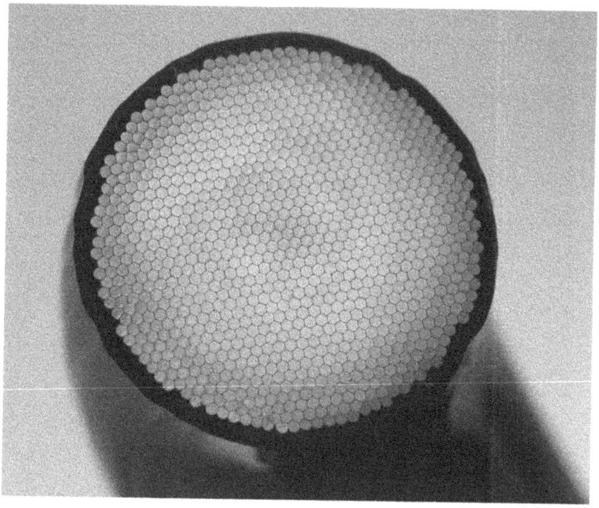

Fig. 5.6 The glass-fibre bundle contained within the larger diameter of an optic tip 'cladding'. The active diameter of the beam profile could be of slightly less than the area of the glass fibre bundle

5.3.2 Consider the Distance/Angulation of the LCU Tip

The irradiance can only equal the radiant exitance when the tip guide is in contact/very close to the restoration surface. Distance from the curing tip to the to the targeted surface will result in loss of energy and irradiance received. A 20%–25% loss of irradiance was measured at 10–11 mm distance from three different LCUs (Fig. 5.7). An angled light guide is a more significant problem as it can reduce the amount of energy delivered. The accessibility of a posterior restoration, especially when located buccally or distally, is challenging. This could affect the potential quality of the restoration as energy delivered is reduced to 33–46% at 45° and is minimal at 25° angulation. Another significant issue with such angulation is the shadow where one wall blocks the light (Fig. 5.7).

5.3.3 Consider Thermal Energy from the LCU and the Polymerization Kinetics

Although LED devices are the most energy-efficient light sources we have, (about 30–40% efficient, compared with 1% for incandescent bulbs) LED chips still produce some heat from the supplied electrical power. Heat energy from LCUs is transferred to the optic tip mainly by non-radiative means such as conduction. This contributes to transient temperature increases [18], depending upon the LED design and exposure duration [19].

During polymerization, C=C bonds convert into C-C bonds which is an exothermic chemical process and thus a source of internal heat generation within the material. As heat is initially generated faster than it can be dissipated, internal temperatures

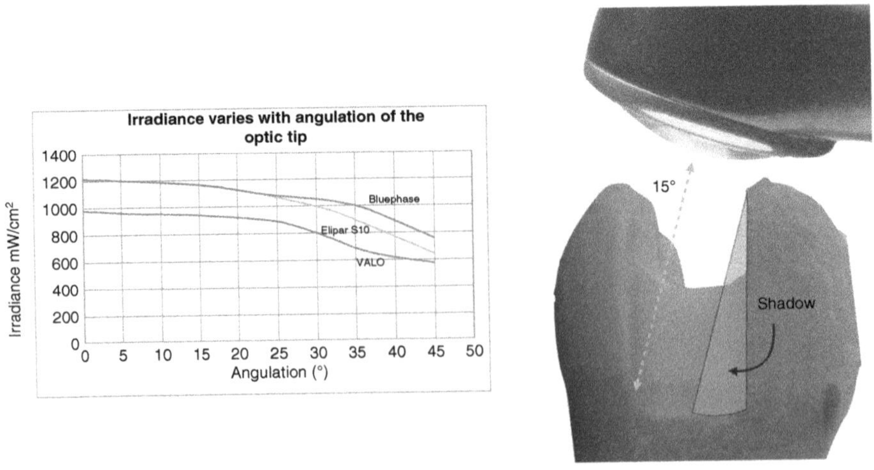

Fig. 5.7 Irradiance can vary with the angulation of the optic tip and also the cavity walls can create an area in shadow

rise to a peak and then diminish. Moderate temperature rises are beneficial to the speed and efficiency of polymerization. However, the clinician must guard against excessive heat generation by avoiding over-irradiation with high-power LEDs [19, 20].

5.4 How Can LCU Performance Be Validated?

Most recent dental innovations concern modified material compositions either to improve properties and performance or to reduce clinical steps. Clinicians may be more focussed upon material steps and neglect awareness of LCU device requirements. For example, many Norwegian general dentists had little knowledge of essential technical specifications of their LCUs. 78% (n = 1313) did not know the irradiance level of their curing light and most did not ensure regular maintenance [21]. This is concerning as restoration quality could potentially be impaired.

The performance of a LED-LCU can be validated by analysis of the emitted light and/or by its effects on a photo-polymerizable resin composite. This can be accomplished either using precision laboratory instrumentation or in the dental clinic using simpler equipment and methods but with reduced quality assurance.

5.4.1 Precision Laboratory Methods

A radiometric measuring device designed specifically for dental LCUs is the MARC-LC™ instrument (BlueLight Analytics Inc., Halifax, Canada). This incorporates a small spectrometer that measures light in the UV and visible spectral range (UV-VIS). The associated software drives the device to record the output spectrum and the irradiance versus time for a pre-set period. The device is calibrated according to—what are known as—*traceable standards*—validated with reference to national and international physical laboratories. The same company measures and certifies LCU devices from leading manufacturers, measuring both radiant output and the resultant beam profile.

Independent laboratories can make similar measurements with UV-VIS spectrometers, referencing to a purchased and calibrated light source [22].

As noted above, the ISO Standard (ISO 10650: 2018) is primarily concerned to establish that radiant emittances *do not exceed* certain limits for three specific wavelength ranges. This Standard does not currently specify any means of measuring beam profiles. However, several papers have been published describing suitable equipment and software. The former includes digital cameras, filters, and a ground-glass diffusing screen from which images of the output beam may be recorded.

Developers of such standards have decided against using any kind of standardized resin composite to check LCU performance since there are so many formulation variables and problems of shelf-life that make the setting of performance limits difficult. Nevertheless, any well-equipped materials science laboratory should have a precision micro-hardness instrument, equipped with a Vickers or Knoop pyramidal diamond indenter. This can be used to study the resultant surface hardness achieved by photo-curing. The specific surfaces that can be measured are as follows:

5.4.1.1 Top and Bottom Hardness

When a clinician photo-cures a resin composite in an occlusal cavity, a hard occlusal surface of the restoration is expected. However, it remains possible that insufficient light has reached the interior and that the lower portion of the restoration may be uncured and soft.

To check this, a suitable plastic or metal mould may be used. For example, a circular hole may be drilled into plastic sheet of either 2 mm or 4 mm thickness. The 4 mm depth may be used for a bulk fill resin composite. The hole ('cavity') may be filled with the composite paste and flat surfaces produced above and below, using matrix strip and glass microscope slides. Following irradiation from the upper or 'occlusal' surface, the hardness can be measured on both the top and bottom surfaces, to give the values: H_T and H_B. These can then be re-expressed to give the *relative bottom hardness*: $\{H_B/H_T\}.100\%$.

Ideally this ratio should be >90%.

In detail, there are several practical variables such as: (a) the type of plastic or metal mould and (b) whether or not a white reflective base is used below the mould.

5.4.1.2 Slotted Moulds to Measure Hardness/Depth Profiles

A more sophisticated mould may be used containing a machined rectangular groove and fitted with a cover plate. The composite paste is placed along the groove and the cover-plate fitted. The composite is then photo-cured from one end. After elapse of, say, 24 h and removal of the cover plate, a series of micro-indents are made at successive distances from the same end. A typical plot of hardness versus depth is shown in Fig. 5.8 [23].

5.4.2 Simpler Measurements in the Dental Clinic

Several hand-help portable radiometers are available for clinical use. Some manufacturers now integrate them with the LCU charging base. These are not high-precision devices but can be useful to check against any sudden deterioration in LCU performance. They give a single numerical reading which is based upon an average of the spectral output. Thus, it is vital to distinguish devices that were intended for use with the older QTH sources from those now available for LED-LCUs. Also, the better devices take into account the exit-diameter of the light guide.

Furthermore, it is possible to estimate the relative top/bottom hardness using the type of plastic mould mentioned above. A sharp probe should not make a significant indentation or scratch on the *lower* surface of the composite. Also, if available, a groove-type mould can be filled with paste to a 'depth' (from the end) exceeding the minimum: say to 6 mm for a bulk fill composite. Following photo-cure from one end of the covered groove, any un-hardened paste may be scraped away. The

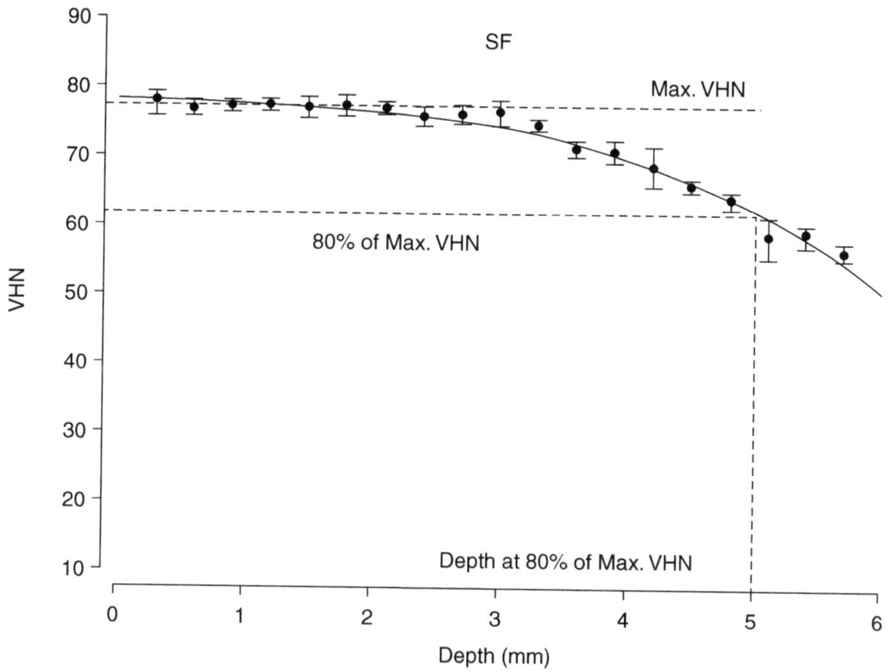

Fig. 5.8 Plot of Vickers hardness number (VHN) versus depth into a bulk-fill material (SF). The depth corresponding to the point where the curve decreases to 80% of the hardness maximum is often taken as the depth of cure [23]

remaining depth has been taken as an estimate of cure-depth, although the ISO 4049 Standard specifies division of this 'raw' value by a factor of two.

It is also possible to place such a specimen in a strong solvent, such as chloroform, to dissolve away uncured material: a good educational experiment.

5.4.3 Developing Photocuring Skills and Good Working Practice

It is important to acquire skills in photo-curing early in the dental school curriculum. This should demonstrate how small movement of the curing light tip can significantly reduce the irradiance. As in any psychomotor skills training, students must understand the importance of the position and stability of the light guide to achieve an efficient polymerization and—thereby—produce a good quality restoration.

Above all, the key necessity is for dentists to check their equipment periodically and to investigate further if there are signs of deteriorating performance. It is good to establish a logbook in which the findings of regular checks are recorded and signed off and to create suitable labels for direct placement on the equipment (Fig. 5.9).

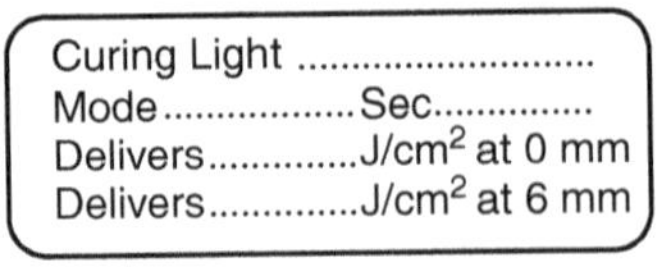

Fig. 5.9 Label for monitoring energy delivered by a LCU during regular maintenance, at the College of Dentistry, University of Iowa. (Courtesy: Dr. Steve Armstrong, University of Iowa)

References

1. Dart EC, Nemcek J. British Patent 1 408 265; 1975.
2. Cayless MA, Marsden AM. Tungsten halogen lamps. In: Lamps and lighting. 3rd ed. London: Edward Arnold; 1983. p. 169–82.
3. Round HJ. A note on carborundum. Electr World. 1907;49:308.
4. Schubert EF. Light-emitting diodes. 2nd ed. Cambridge: Cambridge University Press; 2006.
5. Royal Swedish Academy of Sciences. Scientific background on the Nobel prize in physics 2014: efficient blue light-emitting diodes leading to bright and energy-saving white light sources; 2014.
6. Mills RW. Blue light emitting diodes—another method of light curing? Br Dent J. 1995;178:169.
7. Mills RW, Jandt KD, Ashworth SH. Dental composite depth of cure with halogen and blue light emitting diode technology. Br Dent J. 1999;186:388–91.
8. Mills RW, Jandt KD. United States patent US 7,645,056 B1. Koninklijke Philips Electronics NV; 2010.
9. Stahl F, Ashworth SH, Jandt KD, Mills RW. Light emitting diode (LED) polymerisation of composites: flexural properties and polymerisation potential. Biomaterials. 2000;2: 1379–85.
10. Jandt KD, Mills RW, Blackwell GB, Ashworth SH. Depth of cure and compressive strength of composites cured with blue light emitting diodes (LEDs). Dent Mater. 2000;16:41–7.
11. Bennett AW, Watts DC. Performance of two blue light-emitting-diode dental curing units with distance and irradiation time. Dent Mater. 2004;20:72–9.
12. Jandt KD, Mills RW. A brief history of LED photopolymerization. Dent Mater. 2013;29: 605–17.
13. www.lumileds.com.
14. Cao D. Light for use in activating light-activated materials, the light having a plurality of light emitting semiconductor chips emitting light of differing peak wavelengths to provide a wide light spectrum profile. United States patent US 2002/0190659 A1 to Cao Group, Inc.; 2002.
15. International Standard: ISO 10650. Dentistry–powered polymerization activators. 2nd ed. Geneva: ISO; 2018.
16. Watts DC. Reaction kinetics and mechanics in photopolymerized networks. Dent Mater. 2005;21:27–35.
17. https://www.ivoclarvivadent.co.uk/en-uk/p/all/bluephase-powercure.
18. Randolph LD, Palin WM, Watts DC, Genet M, Devaux J, Leloup G, et al. The effect of ultra-fast photopolymerisation of experimental composites on shrinkage stress, network formation and pulpal temperature rise. Dent Mater. 2014;30:1280–9.
19. Kim M-J, Kim RJ-Y, Ferracane J, Lee I-B. Thermographic analysis of the effect of composite type, layering method, and curing light on the temperature rise of photo-cured composites in tooth cavities. Dent Mater. 2017;33:e373–e83.
20. Yang J, Algamaiah H, Watts DC. Spatio-temporal temperature fields generated coronally with bulk-fill resin composites: thermography methods development. Dent Mater. 2021; 37:1237.

21. Kopperud S, Rukke H, Kopperud H, Bruzell E. Light curing procedures–performance, knowledge level and safety awareness among dentists. J Dent. 2017;2017(58):67–73.
22. Shortall AC, Felix CJ, Watts DC. Robust spectrometer-based methods for characterizing radiant excitance of dental LED light curing units. Dent Mater. 2015;31:339–50.
23. Alrahlah A, Silikas N, Watts DC. Post-cure depth of cure in bulk fill resin-composites. Dent Mater. 2014;30:149–54.

Physical and Mechanical Properties of BFC's

6

Gaetano Paolone and Alessandro Vichi

6.1 Introduction

Resin-based composites (RBCs) have advanced significantly in the past few years. Filler type, resin matrix, and initiator systems have frequently been updated to improve the mechanical properties and to decrease polymerization shrinkage stress. The purpose of these improvements is intended to enhance the clinical longevity of RBC restorations, to reduce the complexity of the restorative procedure, and to decrease chairside time. The recent introduction of bulk fill RBCs represents a revolution in restorative dentistry and provides the clinician considerably shorter chairside time. Since their introduction these materials are now used by clinicians as an alternative to conventional resin composite for posterior restorations and for core build-ups [1].

Full body bulk fill resins require a shorter restorative time in posterior teeth than conventional resins. Flowable bulk fill resin composites provide faster treatment options with time when considering capping [2]. Clinically, a reduction in operative time has been considered a positive reason for selecting bulk fill products [3]. For light-cured bulk fill RBCs, insufficient polymerization at increasing depths has been reported in some studies. This limitation might compromise the clinical success of the restorations with the possibility of increased cytotoxicity [4], susceptibility to marginal defects [5, 6], and reduced hardness [7–9].

There is scientific evidence that the degree of conversion of a resin-based material may influence various mechanical properties, such as BFS (biaxial flexural strength) and KHN (Knoop hardness) [10–13].

G. Paolone (✉)
Dental School, IRCCS San Raffaele Hospital, Vita-Salute University, Milan, Italy
e-mail: paolone.gaetano@hsr.it

A. Vichi
Dental Academy, University of Portsmouth, Portsmouth, UK
e-mail: alessandro.vichi@port.ac.uk

J. Sabbagh, R. McConnell (eds.), *Bulk Fill Resin Composites in Dentistry*,
https://doi.org/10.1007/978-3-031-16388-3_6

Data on curing efficiency has also been inconclusive, with some studies reporting depths of cure of more than 4 mm and others describing insufficient curing at 4-mm layers [14–18].

Differences in mechanical properties and depth of cure may be attributed to differences in resin compositions, material translucency, viscosity, filler type, and content [19].

The mechanical properties of bulk fill RBCs have been, in fact, the subject of some debate. While some authors have reported lower mechanical properties than conventional highly filled RBCs, others have reported values close to conventional materials [20–22].

The type of organic matrix, filler size and morphology, monomer type and ratio, and photoinitiation chemistries vary greatly between products [23]. This makes a comparison of the mechanical properties very difficult [23].

6.2 Flexural Strength

Flexural testing is widely used in characterizing RBCs since it determines both flexural (elastic) modulus and strength and is an important property for restorative materials used in high-stress-bearing areas [24, 25]. Flexural modulus describes the stiffness of RBCs, whereas flexural strength represents the maximum stress that RBCs can be subjected to prior to failure. Elastic modulus is an indicator of stiffness and an important factor affecting shrinkage stress of resin-based composites [26]. Significant relationships between the modulus and stress have been reported by several researchers [27–30].

A lower Young's modulus may allow stress dissipation during the polymerization process, thus reducing the stress when bigger increments are used [10, 31–34].

Certain low-viscosity bulk fill RBCs (flowable) have a modulus of elasticity (and hardness) considerably below the mean values measured for regular nano-hybrid and micro-hybrid RBCs. For this reason, manufacturers recommend covering flowable bulk fill RBC restoration with a capping layer made of regular RBCs [21].

The variation between the flexural properties of various RBCs is useful for different clinical situations [35, 36]. For example, in class I, II, III, and IV cavities, RBCs with high flexural properties are usually selected to minimize fracture or deformation under the high occlusal forces, while in class V cavities, RBCs having low flexural modulus are preferred, as they can flex with the teeth during function and parafunction, which in turn reduces the stresses at the adhesive interface and decreases the chances of debonding [35, 37]. In fact, with their greater flexibility, bulk fill flowable RBCs are preferred over full body bulk fill restorative or conventional materials in deep class V cavities, as they appear to offer better marginal adaptation [38].

The flexural modulus of the bulk fill flowable RBCs is lower than for full body bulk fill restorative or conventional resin composites [33, 39]. A material with a low modulus of elasticity, particularly when placed in load-bearing areas, will result in higher deformability under masticatory stresses and a reduction of wear resistance.

Over time this will cause catastrophic failure of the restoration [21, 40]. Testing of the flexural properties of the different categories of bulk fill materials and those from the different manufacturers are both material and specimen conditioning dependent as confirmed by several authors [39, 41].

The decrease in BFS (biaxial flexural strength) of bulk fill materials with depth was seen to be highly product-dependent [42].

The flexural strength of full body/high-viscosity bulk fill is higher than the limit of 80 MPa established in ISO 4049/2009 for polymer-based restorative materials indicated for restorations involving occlusal surfaces [43, 44]. Bulk fill restorative RBCs (full body) are generally stiffer than bulk fill flowable and conventional counterparts. This may be attributed to the similar or higher filler content of the bulk fill restoratives in comparison to the other RBCs [45–47]. Some authors have reported no correlation between the elastic modulus and filler content for high-viscosity composites, but a strong correlation is generally noted for low-viscosity resins. The low correlation between high-viscosity composites may occur because they present a relatively lower elastic modulus when compared to their filler content [48, 49]. Some flowable and packable resin composites have demonstrated an increase in the elastic modulus 12 h after irradiation due to post-irradiation polymerization [27, 50]. Furthermore, there is an increase in the polymerization stress and the elastic modulus for many bulk fill resin composites after irradiation as they develop a major part of their stiffness within 1 h [51]. The correlation between the degree of conversion and elastic modulus for bulk fill composites is controversial. Some authors have reported that there is no correlation between the degree of conversion and elastic modulus [16].

6.3 Microhardness and Wear of Bulk Fill RBCs

Assessment of a material's hardness is often used by RBCs researchers. Microhardness allows an understanding of the mechanical properties of the composite surfaces [52]. Furthermore, there is a strong relationship between microhardness and elastic modulus values, depth of cure, and polymerization shrinkage [53]. Microhardness is used, in fact, as an indirect measurement of the extent of polymerization of a specific composite material [54, 55], due to its proven correlation with the degree of conversion [56, 57].

According to Watts and others, an acceptable curing depth is achieved if the bottom hardness corresponds to at least 80% of the top surface hardness [58]. The decrease in microhardness of bulk fill materials with depth was also seen to be highly product-dependent, with some materials demonstrating similar hardness values at 1 and 4 mm depth levels [42]. Alrahlah et al. [17], using Vickers hardness profiles, determined that the depth of cure of various bulk fill composite materials ranged from 4.14 to 5.03 mm, which confirms the claims of the manufacturers for the tested materials. An increase in microhardness values is generally expected as the filler content increases. This assumption has been confirmed by several authors [14, 20, 59–64].

Flowable Bulk fill resins have lower microhardness because of the low percentage values for load particles. It is therefore always necessary to apply a conventional resin over them [65, 66].

Papadogiannis et al. reported that the use of a capping layer is mandatory to achieve higher creep resistance [67]. High-viscosity (full body) bulk fill RBCs generally have higher filler content and can be used to cover the softer flowable RBCs or they can be used to fill the entire restorations as they have better wear resistance and improved mechanical properties [44, 68]. Besides the filler size and shape, the hardness of the fillers, the strength of the bond between the inorganic content and polymer matrix, and the light-curing of the RBC can also affect wear resistance [69].

Melo et al. compared conventional resin composites using incremental fill technique and bulk fill RBCs. The conventional composites presented good physical properties, but the bulk fill composites showed better results for surface hardness and solubility at the bottom surface [70].

High variability in the results could be detected for the microhardness test, even among high-viscosity bulk fill resin composites. This may be explained by the lower elastic modulus observed for some of the bulk fill RBCs, generally associated with a differences in filler contents and matrix [21, 61, 62, 71].

Camassari et al. evaluated the physical–mechanical properties of several bulk fill materials submitted to biodegradation by oral biofilm (S. Mutans). Increased roughness and reduced hardness and gloss of all the evaluated composites were reported. The biodegradation induced by *S. mutans* negatively affected mechanical and surface properties. It is therefore mandatory to select the proper restorative material and to advice the patient about the importance of good oral hygiene techniques to maintain the esthetics and longevity of RBC restorations [72].

6.4 Diametral Tensile Strength (DTS)

The diametral compression test may also be used to measure strength [73]. However, the results of such test should be consciously judged, as sometimes shear and tensile stresses may occur at the same time, determining a different fracture pattern,. Moreover, this test is not defined by standards for dental materials. Al Sunbul et al. reported different DTS values for several bulk fill materials (SDR, Venus bulk Fill, Tetric Evoceram Bulk fill, Ever X Posterior) [74]. They reported that the differences at baseline were also confirmed after aging in water and in food simulating solvents: ethanol and methyl ethyl ketone. The authors did not report a correlation between filler loading and mechanical properties. They did not report a correlation between DTS and hardness. Conversely Medeiros et al. reported a strong correlation among these two properties [75].

6.5 Water Sorption

Water sorption is crucial in determining clinical success. Although resin composite is considered in general as a stable material that can accomplish several years of clinical service, the presence of polymer networks determines a certain degree of moisture sorption. Water sorption has a negative effect on the restorative material by contributing to lower/weaken mechanical properties, reduce wear resistance, and affect discoloration.

The effect of water sorption on the resin composite behavior is influenced by several factors, such as the composition of the polymer matrix, the type and content of the filler, and the size and shape of filler particles [76].

Janda et al. [77] investigated water sorption and solubility differences between various types of dental resin composites and reported that the correlation between water sorption and filler load was significant. The lowest water sorption values were found in the composite with the highest filler load. Sorption into a polymer can be explained by two theories: the free volume theory, and the interaction theory [78]. The free volume theory involves solvent absorption through voids in the polymer, while in the interaction theory, water binds to specific ionic groups of the polymer chain depending on their water affinity [79]. Water sorption may decrease the longevity of a RBC resin by expanding and plasticizing its components, causing the hydrolysis of the silane coupling agents. The expansion is undesirable because of the potential stress inducing microcracks or even macrocracks in restored teeth [80]. Bis-GMA-based resin matrix presents higher water sorption because of its hydrophilicity in respect to other methacrylate monomers, such as UDMA [81]. When Bis-GMA resins are combined with TEGDMA to manage viscosity, water uptake can even increase more [82]. Kalachandra et al. supported this finding reporting that partial substitution of TEGDMA with UDMA comonomer in Bis-GMA/TEGDMA RBCs resulted in decreased water absorption [83].

Alshali et al. reported higher sorption values for a conventional flowable (X-Flow, Dentsply Sirona, Kostanz, Germany) compared to a flowable bulk fill (X-tra base, Voco GmbH, Cuxhaven, Germany), the latter showing the lowest values when compared to other bulk fill or conventional nano-hybrid composites [59].

Apart from matrix, fillers play a role in staining susceptibility of RBCs. They are added to increase mechanical properties, to reduce the volume of resin matrix, thus reducing shrinkage and water sorption [84]. Glass fillers do not contribute to the water sorption process but water may get adsorbed onto their surface. The hydrolytic degradation of resin–filler interface bonds can in fact induce the release of unreacted monomers [85], compromising the material biocompatibility [78].

Water sorption depends therefore on material's filler load, with flowable, and low-viscosity bulk fill showing a higher degree, rather than on the polymerization extent characteristic of bulk fill materials. In other words, it is not the fact of being a bulk fill that determines the level of water sorption, rather the viscosity.

6.6 Differences in Mechanical Properties Between Flowable, Full Body, and Fiber-Reinforced Bulk Fill Composites

Differences in mechanical properties have been reported between flowable, full body, and fiber-reinforced bulk fill materials. Because of their poor mechanical properties the use of low-viscosity bulk fill composite is not recommended in

Table 6.1 A comparison of the mechanical properties of different classes of restorative materials

	Conventional flowable RBC	Low-viscosity BF	Fiber-reinforced BF	High-viscosity BF	Conventional RBC
Young modulus [18, 88]	+		++	+++	++++
Vicker hardness [18, 65, 66]	+	++	+++	++++	+++++
Indentation modulus [18]	+			++	+++
Fracture toughness [88]			++	+	
Flexural strength [88]			+	+	

situations where high mechanical stress is present, such as in direct contact with occlusal loads [86, 87]. Previous findings showed that Young modulus, Vickers hardness, and Indentation modulus classify some bulk fill materials (SureFil SDR, Venus Bulk Fill, and Filtek Bulk Fill) as between hybrid and flowable composites [18]. The poor mechanical properties of flowable bulk fill composites highlights the need of coverage with a conventional RBC. This capping procedure should be performed to overcome poor surface properties, low esthetics and material degradation [20]. Attik et al. reported that fiber-reinforced bulk fill show lower flexural modulus and hardness than full body bulk fills [88]. The authors reported similar flexural strength between these two types of bulk fill materials. This leads to the conclusion that fiber-reinforced bulk fill materials may endure higher strain before being damaged.

Fiber-reinforced materials have significantly higher fracture toughness results, showing the higher toughness established by the fiber reinforcement. These materials may prevent fracture propagation inside the material and are indicated for the restoration of endodontically treated teeth [89]. Fiber-reinforced materials undergo higher stress during polymerization [90].

The mechanical properties of flowable bulk fill composites are generally lower compared with the full body high-viscosity materials, and, at best are comparable to the conventional flowable composite [20, 91] as given in Table 6.1.

6.7 Cytotoxicity

While their physico-mechanical properties, handling characteristics and wear performance have been extensively tested [14, 17, 20, 92–94], scientific data on the biocompatibility of bulk fill composite materials is very limited [95]. Biocompatibility is the ability of materials to coexist with living tissues without causing harm. Non-biocompatible or cytotoxic (i.e., toxic to cells) restorative materials can cause short-term and long-term adverse tissue reactions ranging from postoperative sensitivity to irreversible pulp damage [96]. It has been reported that RBCs alone may contribute to more than 12% of adverse reactions of dental materials [97]. In addition to the leaching of unreacted monomers, cytotoxicity can also be caused by the release of initiators and other additives from the organic resin as well as metal ions from the inorganic fillers. Proper curing of RBCs is important to ensure adequate mechanical properties and biocompatibility [98, 99]. This materials' cytotoxicity has been related to the released residual monomer quantity and type; some studies reported a correlation between this aspect and loss of mass and/or lower conversion degree [100]. Bulk fill RBCs placed with a 4 mm single increment present lower shrinkage stress and higher DOC at this depth; this can be related to the increased translucency and to polymerization modulators [3, 101]. However, a common concern about bulk fill materials is whether the degree of conversion at 4 mm depth is sufficient, which would increase the cytotoxic potential, especially in the case of bulk fill flowable resins with a higher organic matter content [102, 103].

Some authors have concluded that the placement of bulk fill composite materials in contrast to conventional resin composite, in a 4-mm layer thickness could be recommended in terms of both mechanical stability and biocompatibility [104].

Alshali et al. [59] reported that despite the increased increment thickness of bulk fill composites, monomer elution from these materials can be comparable to that of conventional composites, with the rate of elution being dependent on monomer molecular weight and the cross-link density of the polymer [105–107]. While highly cross-linked polymers are more resistant to solvent uptake and swelling, linear polymers provide more space and pathways for diffusion of solvent molecules within the structure [82, 108].

The fact that RBCs are biologically accepted, allergic effects on oral soft tissues have been reported [109]. These are generally due to the dissolution of methacrylate and leaching of its components [110], resulting from masticatory forces and chemical degradation [104]. Conversely, Gonçalves et al. reported no toxic response to gingival fibroblasts for bulk fill RBCs placed at the thickness of 4 mm [31].

Others have investigated potential genotoxic effects emanating from resin-based bulk fill materials. They concluded that none of the tested bulk fill resin composites caused primary DNA damage. The finding that eluates obtained from both the top and bottom composite surface of the tested bulk fill materials did not induce genotoxic effects might be explained by an adequate extent of polymerization of the bulk fill resin composites, even when applied in 4-mm thickness.

An irradiation time of 20 s (at an irradiance of ≈1200 mW/cm^2) might suffice for the bulk fill resin composites to not induce relevant genotoxic effects [104].

6.8 Clinical Significance

According to the properties described above, some clinical considerations can be drawn:

- Flowable bulk fill materials must be capped with a conventional RBC.
- In patients with parafunctional habits, restorative materials with higher mechanical properties should be selected.

- Fiber-reinforced BF could be selected to restore ETT as they reduce fracture propagation.
- Adequate curing of bulk fill materials is mandatory to ensure a correct conversion, increase mechanical properties and to reduce cytotoxicity.

6.9 Conclusions

Bulk fill materials can be inserted and polymerized in large increments, in posterior teeth. Although this is a clinical advantage, clinicians should always be aware of the limitations of the mechanical properties of these materials.

A number of bulk fill materials show lower mechanical properties when compared to highly filled nano-hybrid composites. The use of flowable bulk fill materials for restorations under high occlusal load is subject to caution. It is a critical requirement that flowable materials be veneered or capped with a conventional or full body bulk fill material not only to improve esthetics but to reduce the impact of degradation.

Suitably designed clinical studies are required to avoid the biases observed in in vitro studies to better understand clinical performances of these materials.

References

1. Warangkulkasemkit S, Pumpaluk P. Comparison of physical properties of three commercial composite core build-up materials. Dent Mater J. 2019;38(2):177–81.
2. Bellinaso MD, Soares FZM, de Olivera RR. Do bulk-fill resins decrease the restorative time in posterior teeth? A systematic review and meta-analysis of in vitro studies. J Investig Clin Dent. 2019;10(4):e12463.
3. Benetti AR, Havndrup-Pedersen C, Honoré D, Pedersen MK, Pallesen U. Bulk-fill resin composites: polymerization contraction, depth of cure, and gap formation. Oper Dent. 2015;40(2):190–200.
4. Price RB, Shortall AC, Palin WM. Contemporary issues in light curing. Oper Dent. 2014;39(1):4–14.
5. Frassetto A, Breschi L, Turco G, Marchesi G, Di Lenarda R, Tay FR, et al. Mechanisms of degradation of the hybrid layer in adhesive dentistry and therapeutic agents to improve bond durability—a literature review. Dent Mater. 2016;32(2):e41–53.
6. Ferracane JL, Mitchem JC, Condon JR, Todd R. Wear and marginal breakdown of composites with various degrees of cure. J Dent Res. 1997;76(8):1508–16.
7. Soto-Montero J, Nima G, Rueggeberg FA, Dias C, Giannini M. Influence of multiple peak light-emitting-diode curing unit beam homogenization tips on microhardness of resin composites. Oper Dent. 2020;45(3):327–38.
8. Price RBT, Labrie D, Rueggeberg FA, Sullivan B, Kostylev I, Fahey J. Correlation between the beam profile from a curing light and the microhardness of four resins. Dent Mater. 2014;30(12):1345–57.
9. Uhl A, Mills RW, Jandt KD. Photoinitiator dependent composite depth of cure and Knoop hardness with halogen and LED light curing units. Biomaterials. 2003;24(10):1787–95.
10. Fronza BM, Rueggeberg FA, Braga RR, Mogilevych B, Soares LES, Martin AA, et al. Monomer conversion, microhardness, internal marginal adaptation, and shrinkage stress of bulk-fill resin composites. Dent Mater. 2015;31(12):1542–51.

11. Fronza BM, Ayres A, Pacheco RR, Rueggeberg FA, Dias C, Giannini M. Characterization of inorganic filler content, mechanical properties, and light transmission of bulk-fill resin composites. Oper Dent. 2017;42(4):445–55.
12. Rueggeberg FA, Cole MA, Looney SW, Vickers A, Swift EJ. Comparison of manufacturer-recommended exposure durations with those determined using biaxial flexure strength and scraped composite thickness among a variety of light-curing units. J Esthet Restor Dent. 2009;21(1):43–61.
13. Bouschlicher MR, Rueggeberg FA, Wilson BM. Correlation of bottom-to-top surface micro-hardness and conversion ratios for a variety of resin composite compositions. Oper Dent. 2004;29(6):698–704.
14. Bucuta S, Ilie N. Light transmittance and micro-mechanical properties of bulk fill vs. conventional resin based composites. Clin Oral Investig. 2014;18(8):1991–2000.
15. Garcia D, Yaman P, Dennison J, Neiva G. Polymerization shrinkage and depth of cure of bulk fill flowable composite resins. Oper Dent. 2014 Aug;39(4):441–8.
16. Czasch P, Ilie N. In vitro comparison of mechanical properties and degree of cure of bulk fill composites. Clin Oral Investig. 2013;17(1):227–35.
17. Alrahlah A, Silikas N, Watts DC. Post-cure depth of cure of bulk fill dental resin-composites. Dent Mater. 2014;30(2):149–54.
18. Ilie N, Keßler A, Durner J. Influence of various irradiation processes on the mechanical properties and polymerisation kinetics of bulk-fill resin based composites. J Dent. 2013;41(8):695–702.
19. Jang J-H, Park S-H, Hwang I-N. Polymerization shrinkage and depth of cure of bulk-fill resin composites and highly filled flowable resin. Oper Dent. 2015;40(2):172–80.
20. Leprince JG, Palin WM, Vanacker J, Sabbagh J, Devaux J, Leloup G. Physico-mechanical characteristics of commercially available bulk-fill composites. J Dent. 2014;42(8):993–1000.
21. Ilie N, Bucuta S, Draenert M. Bulk-fill resin-based composites: an in vitro assessment of their mechanical performance. Oper Dent. 2013;38(6):618–25.
22. El Gezawi M, Kaisarly D, Al-Saleh H, ArRejaie A, Al-Harbi F, Kunzelmann KH. Degradation potential of bulk versus incrementally applied and indirect composites: color, microhardness, and surface deterioration. Oper Dent. 2016;41(6):e195–208.
23. Leprince J, Palin WM, Mullier T, Devaux J, Vreven J, Leloup G. Investigating filler morphology and mechanical properties of new low-shrinkage resin composite types. J Oral Rehabil. 2010;37(5):364–76.
24. Paolone MG, Kaitsas R, Paolone G, Kaitsas V. Lingual orthodontics and forced eruption: a means for osseous and tissue regeneration. Prog Orthod. 2008;9(2):46–57.
25. Heintze SD, Zimmerli B. Relevance of in vitro tests of adhesive and composite dental materials, a review in 3 parts. Part 1: approval requirements and standardized testing of composite materials according to ISO specifications. Schweiz Monatsschr Zahnmed. 2011;121(9):804–16.
26. Braga RR, Ballester RY, Ferracane JL. Factors involved in the development of polymerization shrinkage stress in resin-composites: a systematic review. Dent Mater. 2005;21(10):962–70.
27. Yamamoto T, Hanabusa M, Momoi Y, Sakaguchi RL. Polymerization stress of dental resin composite continues to develop 12 hours after irradiation. J Esthet Restor Dent. 2015;27(1):44–54.
28. Condon JR, Ferracane JL. Assessing the effect of composite formulation on polymerization stress. J Am Dent Assoc. 2000;131(4):497–503.
29. Calheiros FC, Braga RR, Kawano Y, Ballester RY. Relationship between contraction stress and degree of conversion in restorative composites. Dent Mater. 2004;20(10):939–46.
30. Feng L, Suh BI. A mechanism on why slower polymerization of a dental composite produces lower contraction stress. J Biomed Mater Res B Appl Biomater. 2006;78(1):63–9.
31. Gonçalves F, de Paiva CLM, Rodrigues-Júnior EC, Costa FV, Marques PA, Francci CE, et al. A comparative study of bulk-fill composites: degree of conversion, post-gel shrinkage and cytotoxicity. Braz Oral Res. 2018;32:e17.

32. Ferracane JL. Resin-based composite performance: are there some things we can't predict? Dent Mater. 2013;29(1):51–8.
33. Jung JH, Park SH. Comparison of polymerization shrinkage, physical properties, and marginal adaptation of Flowable and restorative bulk fill resin-based composites. Oper Dent. 2017;42(4):375–86.
34. Prager M, Pierce M, Atria PJ, Sampaio C, Cáceres E, Wolff M, et al. Assessment of cuspal deflection and volumetric shrinkage of different bulk fill composites using non-contact phase microscopy and micro-computed tomography. Dent Mater J. 2018;37(3):393–9.
35. Yap AUJ, Chandra SP, Chung SM, Lim CT. Changes in flexural properties of composite restoratives after aging in water. Oper Dent. 2002;27(5):468–74.
36. Rodrigues Junior SA, Zanchi CH, de Carvalho RV, Demarco FF. Flexural strength and modulus of elasticity of different types of resin-based composites. Braz Oral Res. 2007;21(1):16–21.
37. Pontes LF, Alves EB, Alves BP, Ballester RY, Dias CGBT, Silva CM. Mechanical properties of nanofilled and microhybrid composites cured by different light polymerization modes. Gen Dent. 2013;61(3):30–3.
38. Szesz A, Parreiras S, Martini E, Reis A, Loguercio A. Effect of flowable composites on the clinical performance of non-carious cervical lesions: a systematic review and meta-analysis. J Dent. 2017;65:11–21.
39. Eweis AH, Yap AU, Yahya NA. Comparison of flexural properties of bulk-fill restorative/flowable composites and their conventional counterparts. Oper Dent. 2020;45(1):41–51.
40. Ferracane JL. Resin composite—state of the art. Dent Mater. 2011;27(1):29.
41. Shibasaki S, Takamizawa T, Nojiri K, Imai A, Tsujimoto A, Endo H, et al. Polymerization behavior and mechanical properties of high-viscosity bulk fill and low shrinkage resin composites. Oper Dent. 2017;42(6):E177–87.
42. de Mendonça BC, Soto-Montero JR, de Castro EF, Pecorari VGA, Rueggeberg FA, Giannini M. Flexural strength and microhardness of bulk-fill restorative materials. J Esthet Restor Dent. 2021;33(4):628–35.
43. Paolone G, Breschi L. Restauri diretti in composito: Le potenzialità di un sistema composito universale. Dent Cadmos. 2017;85(5):306–10.
44. Goracci C, Cadenaro M, Fontanive L, Giangrosso G, Juloski J, Vichi A, et al. Polymerization efficiency and flexural strength of low-stress restorative composites. Dent Mater. 2014;30(6):688–94.
45. Ilie N, Rencz A, Hickel R. Investigations towards nano-hybrid resin-based composites. Clin Oral Investig. 2013;17(1):185–93.
46. Ilie N, Hickel R. Investigations on mechanical behaviour of dental composites. Clin Oral Investig. 2009;13(4):427–38.
47. Masouras K, Silikas N, Watts DC. Correlation of filler content and elastic properties of resin-composites. Dent Mater. 2008;24(7):932–9.
48. Kalliecharan D, Germscheid W, Price RB, Stansbury J, Labrie D. Shrinkage stress kinetics of bulk fill resin-based composites at tooth temperature and long time. Dent Mater. 2016;32(11):1322–31.
49. Al Sunbul H, Silikas N, Watts DC. Polymerization shrinkage kinetics and shrinkage-stress in dental resin-composites. Dent Mater. 2016;32(8):998–1006.
50. Helvatjoglu-Antoniades M, Papadogiannis Y, Lakes RS, Dionysopoulos P, Papadogiannis D. Dynamic and static elastic moduli of packable and flowable composite resins and their development after initial photo curing. Dent Mater. 2006;22(5):450–9.
51. Yamamoto T, Hanabusa M, Kimura S, Momoi Y, Hayakawa T. Changes in polymerization stress and elastic modulus of bulk-fill resin composites for 24 hours after irradiation. Dent Mater J. 2018;37(1):87–94.
52. Pieniak D, Niewczas AM, Walczak M, Zamościńska J. Influence of photopolymerization parameters on the mechanical properties of polymer-ceramic composites applied in the conservative dentistry. Acta Bioeng Biomech. 2014;16(3):29–35.
53. Li J, Li H, Fok ASL, Watts DC. Multiple correlations of material parameters of light-cured dental composites. Dent Mater. 2009;25(7):829–36.

54. Tauböck TT, Oberlin H, Buchalla W, Roos M, Attin T. Comparing the effectiveness of self-curing and light curing in polymerization of dual-cured core buildup materials. J Am Dent Assoc. 2011;142(8):950–6.
55. Tauböck TT, Buchalla W, Hiltebrand U, Roos M, Krejci I, Attin T. Influence of the interaction of light- and self-polymerization on subsurface hardening of a dual-cured core build-up resin composite. Acta Odontol Scand. 2011;69(1):41–7.
56. Rueggeberg FA, Craig RG. Correlation of parameters used to estimate monomer conversion in a light-cured composite. J Dent Res. 1988;67(6):932–7.
57. Price RB, Whalen JM, Price TB, Felix CM, Fahey J. The effect of specimen temperature on the polymerization of a resin-composite. Dent Mater. 2011;27(10):983–9.
58. Watts DC, Amer O, Combe EC. Characteristics of visible-light-activated composite systems. Br Dent J. 1984;156(6):209–15.
59. Alshali RZ, Salim NA, Sung R, Satterthwaite JD, Silikas N. Analysis of long-term monomer elution from bulk-fill and conventional resin-composites using high performance liquid chromatography. Dent Mater. 2015;31(12):1587–98.
60. Rodriguez A, Yaman P, Dennison J, Garcia D. Effect of light-curing exposure time, shade, and thickness on the depth of cure of bulk fill composites. Oper Dent. 2017;42(5):505–13.
61. Tekin TH, Kantürk Figen A, Yılmaz Atalı P, Coşkuner Filiz B, Pişkin MB. Full in-vitro analyses of new-generation bulk fill dental composites cured by halogen light. Mater Sci Eng C Mater Biol Appl. 2017;77:436–45.
62. Son S-A, Park J-K, Seo D-G, Ko C-C, Kwon YH. How light attenuation and filler content affect the microhardness and polymerization shrinkage and translucency of bulk-fill composites? Clin Oral Investig. 2017;21(2):559–65.
63. Miletic V, Pongprueksa P, De Munck J, Brooks NR, Van Meerbeek B. Curing characteristics of flowable and sculptable bulk-fill composites. Clin Oral Investig. 2017;21(4):1201–12.
64. Chung KH, Greener EH. Correlation between degree of conversion, filler concentration and mechanical properties of posterior composite resins. J Oral Rehabil. 1990;17(5):487–94.
65. Garoushi S, Vallittu P, Shinya A, Lassila L. Influence of increment thickness on light transmission, degree of conversion and micro hardness of bulk fill composites. Odontology. 2016;104(3):291–7.
66. Flury S, Peutzfeldt A, Lussi A. Influence of increment thickness on microhardness and dentin bond strength of bulk fill resin composites. Dent Mater. 2014;30(10):1104–12.
67. Papadogiannis D, Tolidis K, Gerasimou P, Lakes R, Papadogiannis Y. Viscoelastic properties, creep behavior and degree of conversion of bulk fill composite resins. Dent Mater. 2015;31(12):1533–41.
68. Van Ende A, De Munck J, Lise DP, Van Meerbeek B. Bulk-fill composites: a review of the current literature. J Adhes Dent. 2017;19(2):95–109.
69. Ilie N, Hilton TJ, Heintze SD, Hickel R, Watts DC, Silikas N, et al. Academy of dental materials guidance-resin composites: part I-mechanical properties. Dent Mater. 2017;33(8):880–94.
70. Melo RA, SL BAD, GAS B, Galvão MR, de Assunção IV, Souza RO, et al. Morphochemical characterization, microhardness, water sorption, and solubility of regular viscosity bulk fill and traditional composite resins. Microsc Res Tech. 2019;82(9):1500–6.
71. Ilie N, Stark K. Effect of different curing protocols on the mechanical properties of low-viscosity bulk-fill composites. Clin Oral Investig. 2015;19(2):271–9.
72. Camassari JR, Correr-Sobrinho L, Correr AB, Puppin-Rontani J, Stipp RN, Puppin-Rontani RM, et al. Physical-mechanical properties of bulk fill composites submitted to biodegradation by Streptococcus mutans. Braz Dent J. 2020;31(4):431–9.
73. Carneiro FLLB, Barcellos A. Concrete tensile strength, Bulletin no. 13, Union of testing and research laboratories for materials and structures, Paris, France; 1953. pp. 97–123.
74. Sunbul HA, Silikas N, Watts DC. Surface and bulk properties of dental resin-composites after solvent storage. Dent Mater. 2016;32(8):987–97.
75. Medeiros IS, Gomes MN, Loguercio AD, Filho LER. Diametral tensile strength and Vickers hardness of a composite after storage in different solutions. J Oral Sci. 2007;49(1):61–6.

76. Alshali RZ, Salim NA, Satterthwaite JD, Silikas N. Long-term sorption and solubility of bulk-fill and conventional resin-composites in water and artificial saliva. J Dent. 2015;43(12):1511–8.
77. Janda R, Roulet J-F, Latta M, Rüttermann S. Water sorption and solubility of contemporary resin-based filling materials. J Biomed Mater Res B Appl Biomater. 2007;82(2):545–51.
78. Wei Y, Silikas N, Zhang Z, Watts DC. Diffusion and concurrent solubility of self-adhering and new resin-matrix composites during water sorption/desorption cycles. Dent Mater. 2011;27(2):197–205.
79. Chaves LP, Graciano FMO, Bim Júnior O, do Vale Pedreira APR, Manso AP, Wang L. Water interaction with dental luting cements by means of sorption and solubility. Braz Dent Sci. 2012;15:29–35.
80. Sideridou ID, Vouvoudi EC, Adamidou EA. Dynamic mechanical thermal properties of the dental light-cured nanohybrid composite Kalore, GC: effect of various food/oral simulating liquids. Dent Mater. 2015;31(2):154–61.
81. Bagheri R, Burrow MF, Tyas M. Influence of food-simulating solutions and surface finish on susceptibility to staining of aesthetic restorative materials. J Dent. 2005;33(5):389–98.
82. Ferracane JL. Hygroscopic and hydrolytic effects in dental polymer networks. Dent Mater. 2006;22(3):211.
83. Kalachandra S, Turner DT. Water sorption of polymethacrylate networks: bis-GMA/TEGDM copolymers. J Biomed Mater Res. 1987;21(3):329–38.
84. Bociong K, Szczesio A, Sokolowski K, Domarecka M, Sokolowski J, Krasowski M, et al. The influence of water sorption of dental light-cured composites on shrinkage stress. Materials (Basel). 2017;10(10):E1142.
85. Yiu CKY, King NM, Pashley DH, Suh BI, Carvalho RM, Carrilho MRO, et al. Effect of resin hydrophilicity and water storage on resin strength. Biomaterials. 2004;25(26):5789–96.
86. El-Safty S, Akhtar R, Silikas N, Watts DC. Nanomechanical properties of dental resin-composites. Dent Mater. 2012;28(12):1292–300.
87. Ilie N, Hickel R. Investigations on a methacrylate-based flowable composite based on the SDR™ technology. Dent Mater. 2011;27(4):348–55.
88. Attik N, Colon P, Gauthier R, Chevalier C, Grosgogeat B, Abouelleil H. Comparison of physical and biological properties of a flowable fiber reinforced and bulk filling composites. Dent Mater. 2022;38(2):e19–30.
89. Eapen AM, Amirtharaj LV, Sanjeev K, Mahalaxmi S. Fracture resistance of endodontically treated teeth restored with 2 different fiber-reinforced composite and 2 conventional composite resin core buildup materials: an in vitro study. J Endod. 2017;43(9):1499–504.
90. Shouha PSR, Ellakwa AE. Effect of short glass fibers on the polymerization shrinkage stress of dental composite. J Biomed Mater Res B Appl Biomater. 2017;105(7):1930–7.
91. Osiewicz MA, Werner A, Roeters FJM, Kleverlaan CJ. Wear of bulk-fill resin composites. Dent Mater. 2021;S0109-5641(21):00473–5.
92. Petrovic LM, Zorica DM, Stojanac IL, Krstonosic VS, Hadnadjev MS, Atanackovic TM. A model of the viscoelastic behavior of flowable resin composites prior to setting. Dent Mater. 2013;29(9):929–34.
93. Barkmeier WW, Takamizawa T, Erickson RL, Tsujimoto A, Latta M, Miyazaki M. Localized and generalized simulated wear of resin composites. Oper Dent. 2015;40(3):322–35.
94. Tauböck TT, Tarle Z, Marovic D, Attin T. Pre-heating of high-viscosity bulk-fill resin composites: effects on shrinkage force and monomer conversion. J Dent. 2015;43(11):1358–64.
95. Toh WS, Yap AUJ, Lim SY. In vitro biocompatibility of contemporary bulk-fill composites. Oper Dent. 2015;40(6):644–52.
96. Geurtsen W. Biocompatibility of resin-modified filling materials. Crit Rev Oral Biol Med. 2000;11(3):333–55.
97. Scott A, Egner W, Gawkrodger DJ, Hatton PV, Sherriff M, van Noort R, et al. The national survey of adverse reactions to dental materials in the UK: a preliminary study by the UK adverse reactions reporting project. Br Dent J. 2004;196(8):471–7; discussion 465.

98. Baharav H, Brosh T, Pilo R, Cardash H. Effect of irradiation time on tensile properties of stiffness and strength of composites. J Prosthet Dent. 1997;77(5):471–4.
99. Caughman WF, Caughman GB, Shiflett RA, Rueggeberg F, Schuster GS. Correlation of cytotoxicity, filler loading and curing time of dental composites. Biomaterials. 1991;12(8):737–40.
100. Salehi S, Gwinner F, Mitchell JC, Pfeifer C, Ferracane JL. Cytotoxicity of resin composites containing bioactive glass fillers. Dent Mater. 2015;31(2):195–203.
101. Marovic D, Tauböck TT, Attin T, Panduric V, Tarle Z. Monomer conversion and shrinkage force kinetics of low-viscosity bulk-fill resin composites. Acta Odontol Scand. 2015;73(6):474–80.
102. Furness A, Tadros MY, Looney SW, Rueggeberg FA. Effect of bulk/incremental fill on internal gap formation of bulk-fill composites. J Dent. 2014;42(4):439–49.
103. Jan Y-D, Lee B-S, Lin C-P, Tseng W-Y. Biocompatibility and cytotoxicity of two novel low-shrinkage dental resin matrices. J Formos Med Assoc. 2014;113(6):349–55.
104. Tauböck TT, Marovic D, Zeljezic D, Steingruber AD, Attin T, Tarle Z. Genotoxic potential of dental bulk-fill resin composites. Dent Mater. 2017;33(7):788–95.
105. Ferracane JL. Elution of leachable components from composites. J Oral Rehabil. 1994;21(4):441–52.
106. Durner J, Obermaier J, Draenert M, Ilie N. Correlation of the degree of conversion with the amount of elutable substances in nano-hybrid dental composites. Dent Mater. 2012;28(11):1146–53.
107. Benetti AR, Asmussen E, Munksgaard EC, Dewaele M, Peutzfeldt A, Leloup G, et al. Softening and elution of monomers in ethanol. Dent Mater. 2009;25(8):1007–13.
108. Cavalcante LM, Schneider LFJ, Silikas N, Watts DC. Surface integrity of solvent-challenged ormocer-matrix composite. Dent Mater. 2011;27(2):173–9.
109. Sevkusic M, Schuster L, Rothmund L, Dettinger K, Maier M, Hickel R, et al. The elution and breakdown behavior of constituents from various light-cured composites. Dent Mater. 2014;30(6):619–31.
110. Darmani H, Al-Hiyasat AS, Milhem MM. Cytotoxicity of dental composites and their leached components. Quintessence Int. 2007;38(9):789–95.

Short Fiber Based Filling Composites

7

Sufyan Garoushi, Filip Keulemans, Lippo Lassila, and Pekka K. Vallittu

7.1 Introduction

Direct conventional resin composite restorations, i.e., particulate filler resin composite (PFC) restorations are a routine approach of treating lost tooth structure conservatively. Beside the ability to bond to hard tooth tissues, mediated by adhesive systems, they feature the advantage of natural shade and are less expensive compared with cast gold and ceramic indirect restorations [1]. The use of resin composites has increased tremendously during the last two decades. Today, resin composites are selected on a regular basis for direct (bulk fill or layered) and laboratory made posterior restorations, as an extension to their original indication, which was limited to direct restorations in anterior teeth. Their use has been widened not only to the posterior intra-coronal area, but also to extra-coronal restorations [2]. In addition, resin composites are used for the fabrication of resin-bonded fixed dental prostheses (RBFDP) following the introduction of fiber-reinforced composites (FRC). However, inadequate material properties limited the success of resin composite restorations in high stress-bearing areas [3, 4]. Resin composites were introduced to the dental community in the 1960s [5]. Since then, significant material improvements have been introduced. However, resin composite still suffers from a lack of mechanical properties and polymerization shrinkage. Resin composite restorations have shown good overall clinical performance in small and medium sized posterior

S. Garoushi (✉) · F. Keulemans · L. Lassila
Department of Biomaterials Science and Turku Clinical Biomaterials Center–TCBC Institute of Dentistry, University of Turku, Turku, Finland
e-mail: sufgar@utu.fi; filip.keulemans@utu.fi; lippo.lassila@utu.fi

P. K. Vallittu
Department of Biomaterials Science and Turku Clinical Biomaterials Center–TCBC Institute of Dentistry, University of Turku, Turku, Finland

City of Turku Welfare Division, Oral Health Care, Turku, Finland
e-mail: pekka.vallittu@utu.fi

J. Sabbagh, R. McConnell (eds.), *Bulk Fill Resin Composites in Dentistry*,
https://doi.org/10.1007/978-3-031-16388-3_7

restorations with annual failure rates between 1% and 3% [3, 6]. Secondary caries and fracture are among the most important reasons for clinical failure [6, 7]. Survival of posterior restorations strongly correlates with the size of the restorations. Bernardo et al. reported an increase in annual failure rate from 0.95% for single-surface restorations to 9.43% for four or more surface restorations [8]. Large restorations were more prone to fracture-related failures resulting in decreased longevity [9, 10]. The higher susceptibility of large resin composite restorations to fracture may be related to the use of glass-ionomer lining material, strength-related properties of the resin composite material itself and patient factors such as bruxism [6, 11]. Besides restoration size the endodontic status of a tooth strongly affects the longevity of resin composite restorations. Clinical studies revealed a decreased longevity for resin composite restorations in endodontically treated teeth, with an increased annual failure rate of 2–12.4% when compared to vital teeth [6, 12]. Furthermore, non-vital teeth are susceptible to unfavorable subgingival cusp fractures [13]. The above-mentioned reasons make the restoration of endodontically treated teeth a true challenge.

It is clear from the literature that contemporary resin composites still demonstrate limitations due to their insufficient mechanical properties when used in large restorations. Due to failures of this kind, it is still controversial, whether restorative resin composites should be used in large high stress-bearing applications such as in direct posterior restorations or core build-ups [3, 14]. The relatively high brittleness and low fracture toughness of current PFCs still hinder their use in these large stress-bearing restorations [15, 16]. Appropriate physical and mechanical properties and satisfactory esthetic are all characteristics that restorative resin composite should achieve.

7.2 Biomimetic Dentistry

Contemporary restorative dentistry uses direct, semi-direct as well as indirect restorations to restore lost tooth tissue with biomimetics as the new driving force. Biomimetic dentistry tries to mimic nature by studying the structure, function and biology of the tooth organ as a model for the design and engineering of new or improved materials and techniques to restore or replace teeth in biomechanically optimal way [17]. From a biomimetic point of view, we strive to replace lost tooth tissue by biomaterials with similar physical properties, especially with reference to fracture toughness, elastic modulus, strength, and thermal expansion coefficient [18, 19]. A well accepted biomimetic restorative approach advocates replacing enamel with feldspathic porcelain or glass ceramic and dentine by conventional PFCs [19, 20]. Although such approach seems effective, there are still relevant mechanical properties, such as fracture toughness, not considered. Fracture toughness of PFC is still lower than that of dentine [1]. Furthermore, the microstructure of PFC does not resemble that of dentine. PFC consists of filler particles embedded in a resin matrix while dentine consists of collagen fibers embedded in a hydroxyapatite matrix. Therefore, dentine should be rather seen as a fiber-reinforced composite. Collagen fibers act as crack stopper and gives dentine unique properties by making it resilient, flexible and tough at the same time. For that reason, improvement might be found when taking advantage of a more dentine-like and high toughness resin composite as dentine replacement.

Extensive research has been conducted to improve the reinforcing phase of restorative PFC in order to increase their suitability for use in high stress-bearing areas. Attempts have been made to change the type of filler or the filler size and their silanization [21–26]. Reinforcing the resin composite with short glass fibers has been one of the most effective approaches among the methods that have been studied [23, 27, 28]. Short fibers enhanced the ability of the material to resist the crack propagation, as well as to reduce the stress intensity at the crack tip from which a crack propagates in an unstable manner. As a consequence, an increased resin composite toughness should be expected. A number of manufacturers have developed short fiber-reinforced composites (SFRCs) which claimed to overcome the weakness of conventional PFC (Table 7.1). However, comparative studies from the literature showed that commercial SFRCs have different properties, structures, and reinforcing capacities [29, 30]. Recent studies showed that millimeter and micrometer scales SFRCs (everX Posterior and everX Flow; GC Corporation) had a significant superior fracture toughness and reinforcing capability when compared to other commercial SFRCs (Alert, NovaPro-Flow, NovaPro-Fill, EasyCore, Build-It and TI-Core) [29, 30]. Based on this, everX

Table 7.1 Short fiber-reinforced composites

Brand	Type	Composition
everX Posterior (GC Corp, Tokyo, Japan)	LC Packable	Bis-GMA, PMMA, TEGDMA, millimeter scale glass fiber filler, barium glass 76 wt%, 57 vol%
everX Flow (GC Corp, Tokyo, Japan)	LC Flowable	Bis-EMA, TEGDMA, UDMA, micrometer scale glass fiber filler, barium glass 70 wt%, 46 vol%
Alert (Jeneric/Pentron, Wallingford, CT, USA)	LC Packable	Bis-GMA, UDMA, TEGDMA, THFMA, silica and micrometer scale glass fiber 84 wt%, 62 vol%
NovaPro Flow (Nanova, Columbia, MO, USA)	LC Flowable	Bis-EMA, UDMA, TEGDMA, Barium silicate, amorphous fumed silica, nanometer scale hydroxyapatite fiber (% NA)
NovaPro Fill (Nanova)	LC Packable	Bis-EMA, UDMA, TEGDMA, Barium silicate, amorphous fumed silica, nanometer scale hydroxyapatite fiber (% NA)
EasyCore (SpofaDental, Markova, Czech Republic)	DC Flowable	Bis-GMA, HDMA, glass fiber
Build-It (Jeneric/Pentron)	DC Flowable	Bis-GMA, UDMA, HDMA, 67.3 wt% Boroaluminosilicate glass and chopped glass fiber
TI-Core (Essential Dental Systems, Hackensack, NJ, USA)	AC Packable	Bis-GMA, titanium and lanthanide reinforced 75 wt%

Bis-GMA bisphenol-A-glycidyl dimethacrylate, *UDMA* urethane dimethacrylate, *TEGDMA* triethylene glycol dimethacrylate, *Bis-EMA* ethoxylated bisphenol-A-dimethacrylate, *THFMA* tetrahydrofurfuryl-2-methacrylate, *PMMA* polymethylmethacrylate, *HDMA* hexanediol dimethacrylate, *LC* light cured, *DC* dual cured, *AC* auto cured, *wt%*, weight percentage, *vol%* volume percentage, *NA* not available

Posterior and everX Flow are the most interesting dentine-replacing materials because of their close resemblance to dentine at the level of microstructure and mechanical properties [18, 31, 32].

7.3 Structure and Properties

Many of the properties of SFRCs are strongly dependent on microstructural parameters such as fiber diameter, fiber length, fiber orientation, fiber loading, and adhesion of fibers to the polymer matrix [33]. For a fiber to act as an effective reinforcement for polymers, stress transfer from the polymer matrix to the fibers is essential [33]. This is achieved by having a fiber length equal to or greater than the critical fiber length and the given fiber aspect ratio in the range of 30–94 [33–35]. Aspect ratio, critical fiber length, and fiber loading are the main factors that could improve or impair the mechanical properties of SFRCs. Aspect ratio is the fiber length to fiber diameter ratio (l/d). It affects the tensile strength and the reinforcing efficiency of the fiber-reinforced material [33]. It should be noted that adhesion of the fibers to the polymer matrix also influences to the critical fiber length. Sufficient adhesion between fiber and matrix provides good load transfer between the two components, which ensures that the load is transferred to the stronger fiber, and this is how the fiber actually works as reinforcement. However, if the adhesion is not strong and if any voids appear between the fiber and the polymer matrix, these voids may act as initial fracture sites in the matrix and facilitate the breakdown of the material [36].

For instance, Alert has fiber length in micrometer scale (20–60 μm) and diameter of 7 μm (Fig. 7.1), while NovaPro composites have fiber diameter in nanometer scale (50–200 nm) and length in range between 100 and 150 μm, which is well below the critical fiber length and desired aspect ratio [30]. This explained the difference in fracture toughness values between the commercial SFRCs. These differences were seen by SEM analysis (Figs. 7.1 and 7.3), which prove that materials

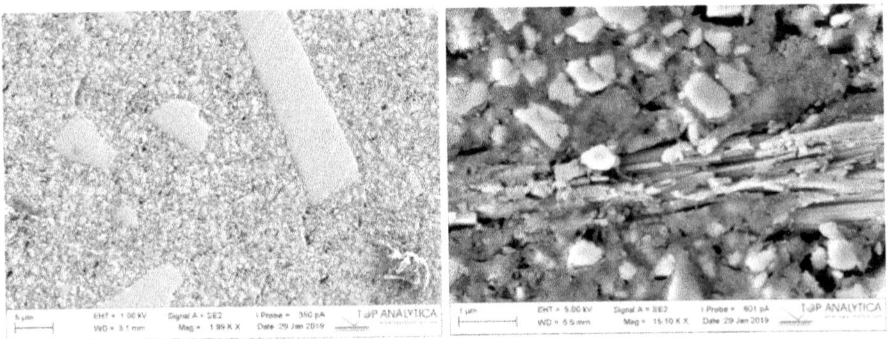

Fig. 7.1 SEM photomicrographs of polished surface of SFRCs showing the micrometer scale fiber in Alert (left side) and nanofiber bundle in the NovaPro Flow (right side)

with different microstructure characteristic and fiber aspect ratio (length and diameter) could differ with regards to physical properties and toughness.

Earlier formulations of SFRC showed a high failure rate due to secondary caries and bulk fracture [37, 38]. Bulk fracture of earlier SFRC formulations was related to sub-optimal reinforcement of the polymer matrix by short fibers. These SFRCs did not fulfill the reinforcing requirements. Aspect ratio and critical fiber length have implications towards fracture toughness (K_{Ic}), a property of major influence on the clinical performance of a material [39]. Fracture toughness of earlier SFRC formulations is much lower than that of dentine [1].

Following this knowledge, a millimeter scales packable SFRC (everX Posterior) was launched in 2013. It consists of a combination of a resin matrix (24 wt%), randomly orientated E-glass fiber (9 wt%) and inorganic particulate fillers (67 wt%) [27, 34]. The resin matrix comprises cross-linked monomers bis-GMA and TEGDMA accompanied with linear PMMA. This combination of resins enables the formation of the semi interpenetrating polymer network (semi-IPN) during the polymerization of the material, which provides good bonding properties and improved toughness of the resin composite [36]. The short, randomly oriented fiber on the other hand, provide an isotropic reinforcing effect when placed in bulk, which means that the strength of the material is independent of the fracture load direction, i.e., it is the same in all directions. Nevertheless, in the origin isotropic SFRC material (3D fiber orientation and fiber reinforcing factor of 0.2) becomes anisotropic and subsequently more biomimetic when applied in incremental layers up to 2 mm thick, due to alignment of fibers in the plane of application (2D fiber orientation and fiber reinforcement factor of 0.38) [33].

In 2019, the flowable version of SFRC (everX Flow) was introduced with the promise of easy handling and better adaptability in limited spaces. It consists of a combination of a resin matrix (30 wt%), randomly orientated glass microfibers (25 wt%) and inorganic silanated particulate fillers (45 wt%) (Fig. 7.2) [40, 41].

The micrometer scale SFRC (everX Flow) had an aspect ratio of more than 30 because the diameter of microglass fibers used was 6 μm and the length in the range

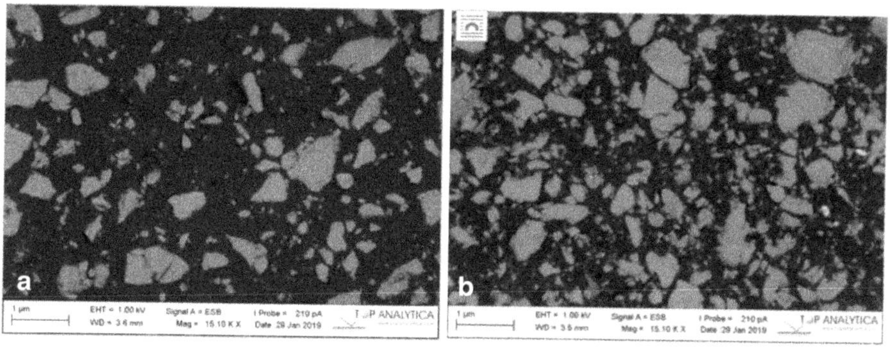

Fig. 7.2 SEM photomicrographs of polished surface of SFRCs (scale bar = 1 μm) showing different filler weight percentages. (**a**) everX Posterior; (**b**) everX Flow

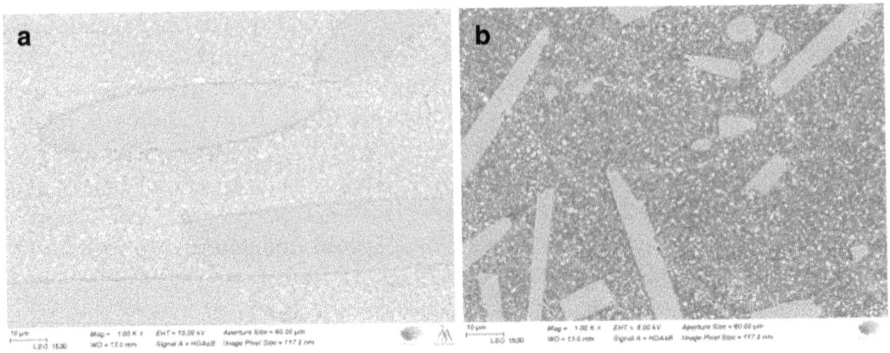

Fig. 7.3 SEM photomicrographs of polished surface of SFRCs (scale bar = 10 μm) showing different fiber diameters. (**a**) everX Posterior; (**b**) everX Flow

of 200–300 μm. everX Posterior had fiber (Ø17 μm) length distribution between 0.3 and 1.5 mm, which is in the range of the reported critical fiber length and desired aspect ratio (Fig. 7.3). It is therefore not surprising that everX Posterior and everX Flow have superior fracture toughness in comparison to all other commercial fiber filled resin composite.

These SFRCs were reported to exhibit improved mechanical properties regarding strength, fracture toughness, fatigue resistance, and polymerization shrinkage and to show a more favorable (repairable) type of failure behavior in comparison to PFCs [27, 28, 35, 40, 42–45]. The use of fiber fillers with a length in the range of the reported critical fiber length and desired aspect ratio, increased K_{Ic} of SFRCs up to 2.6–3.1 MPa $m^{0.5}$ [35, 40, 46, 47] in comparison to 1.2–1.8 MPa $m^{0.5}$ of conventional PFC [48]. Therefore, it can be hypothesized that the replacement of dentine by a high toughness SFRCs can reduce bulk fractures and therefore increase longevity of large resin composite restorations.

There is little evidence comparing bond durability of SFRC to dentine with that of other conventional PFCs [49, 50]. A study by Tsujimoto et al. determined that the relationship between mechanical properties and dentine bond durability of SFRC using universal adhesives showed improvements compared to conventional PFCs [49]. Regardless of adhesive type and etching modes, the ratios of shear fatigue strength and shear bond strength of SFRC were higher than those of conventional PFCs. The authors clarified that superior mechanical properties of SFRC, especially fracture toughness, could improve its bond durability with universal adhesives [49, 50]. Studies have debated if short fibers might have a reinforcing effect on the oxygen-inhibited layer of the adhesive and they emphasized that, with enhanced mechanical properties and bond durability, SFRC might perform better in high stress-bearing situations.

Curiously, SFRCs have the ability to conduct and scatter the curing light better than conventional PFCs and thus it is suitable for use in bulk of 4–5 mm layer thickness [40, 51, 52]. Surface roughness, wear and esthetic related limitations of SFRCs can be overcome by adopting a biomimetic restorative approach, in which dentine is replaced by SFRC and covered by a more wear-resistant PFC [1, 18]. Such

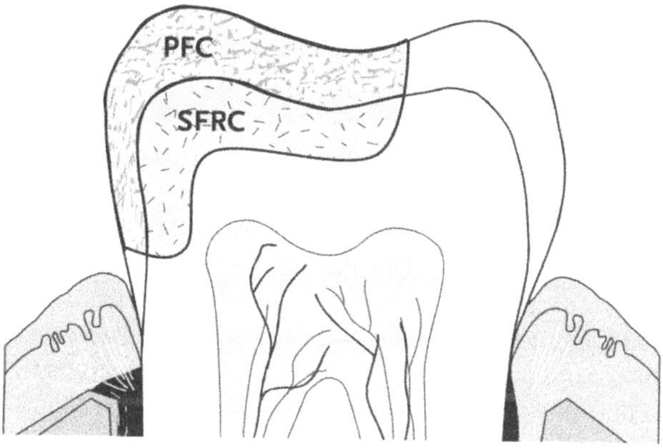

Fig. 7.4 Schematic representation of a direct biomimetic restoration: lost dentine is replaced by high toughness SFRC and covered by a wear-resistant enamel-replacing PFC

approach not only has the benefits of better wear resistance but also increased strength and fatigue resistance. SFRCs are suitable as a bulk base or core foundation and should not be used as final restoration. Although, microfibers filler loading was not seen to be worsening the wear or the gloss of the flowable SFRC (everX Flow) [40, 53]. Clinically, it is widely recommended nowadays to use a layer of composite bulk base (dentine replacing) material in order to improve the esthetic, to reduce the polymerization stress and to develop better mechanical properties [54]. The latter is accomplished by decreasing the tensile stress concentrations at the restoration interface and reducing the cuspal strain [54]. Published clinical results of bilayered restorations (Fig. 7.4) containing SFRC as bulk composite base in high stress-bearing areas have shown good clinical performance. However, the time frame and case numbers for these clinical trials were not of such duration and number as to indicate the long-term suitability of the tested restorations [55–57].

7.4 Benefits of Using SFRCs as Bulk

Bilayered composite structure of SFRC as substructure and PFC as top surface layer (Fig. 7.4) has been evaluated in several in vitro investigations and with different applications [58–63]. SFRC base has already been used to reinforce large direct composites restorations in vital teeth [64–68] as well as in endodontically treated teeth [69–73], as prosthesis infrastructure [74–78], onlay restorations [59, 79], and endodontic post/core foundations [70–73].

The effect of the thickness of the SFRC substructure versus the thickness of the overlaying PFC, static and fatigue load-bearing capacity of materials combination and the interface between SFRC and PFC are among the issues that have been studied [21, 22, 80, 81].

These studies demonstrate that SFRC substructure supports the PFC layer and serve as a crack preventative layer. SFRC substructure's thickness is important, as it influences the failure mode and the crack arresting mechanism. The mechanism of arresting the crack propagation is greatly influenced by the distance between the SFRC substructure and the surface where the stress initiates. The applied SFRC and

PFC layers thickness is extremely important. The ratio between the SFRC base and surface PFC should be an analogue to the dentine and enamel structure. In vitro it was observed that optimal thickness of the veneering PFC composite over the SFRC substructure is around 1 mm [21, 22, 80]. It is important to point out that less benefit is achieved if the layer of SFRC is not sufficiently thick [77, 81]. Other advantages of SFRC-based biomimetic restorations can be seen at the level of the interface between SFRC and PFC [82, 83]. After application of the SFRC layer some fibers are protruding from the surface which can be embedded in the veneering PFC layer and form an interface similar to that found at the dentine-enamel junction (DEJ). At the DEJ, collagen fiber originating from dentine extends into enamel creating a fiber-reinforced connection between enamel and dentine. It is known that the microscopic architecture and the unique mechanical properties of the DEJ acts as a natural crack arrest barrier [84].

Theoretically, the significant advantage of this bilayered or biomimetic restoration is their ability to mimic the natural behavior of enamel and dentine. To the author's knowledge, these SFRCs are the only available resin composites that mimics structurally the dentine at this time.

7.5 Clinical Use of SFRCs

In this series of clinical cases an attempt was made by using SFRCs as bulk base or core material under surface layer of conventional PFC, i.e., direct biomimetic or bilayered composite restorations, in order to improve the load-bearing capacity and clinical longevity of resin-based composite restorations.

7.5.1 Clinical Case: everX Posterior

A 49-year-old male presented with a defective Class II amalgam restoration and a primary carious lesion on a lower second premolar (FDI #45) (Fig. 7.5a). The old restoration was removed using a pear-shaped diamond bur (830 L; Komet) in a high-speed air turbine. Dental dam was placed after opening the cavity, in order to obtain a dry working field. The minimal invasive cavity was cleaned by sandblasting with 50 μm alumina particles. A three-step etch-and-rinse adhesive (Optibond FL, Kerr) was applied according to manufacturer's instructions. The resin composite was placed following an incremental filling technique and interproximal contacts were restored by use of metal sectional matrices in combination with separation rings (V3 matrix and ring, Triodent) (Fig. 7.5b). The centripetal filling technique was adopted to transform the three-surface cavity into a single-surface cavity (Fig. 7.5c): a first 1 mm thick layer of hybrid composite (Filtek Supreme XTE; 3 M ESPE) was placed towards the matrix and the subsequent layers (2 mm thick) of SFRC (everX Posterior; GC) were placed oblique (Fig. 7.5d). The biomimetic restoration was finalized by placing a final 1.5 mm thick increment of hybrid composite at the occlusal surface. Each increment of resin composite was light-cured with an LED-curing unit (The cure; Spring Health Products) for 40 s. Additional

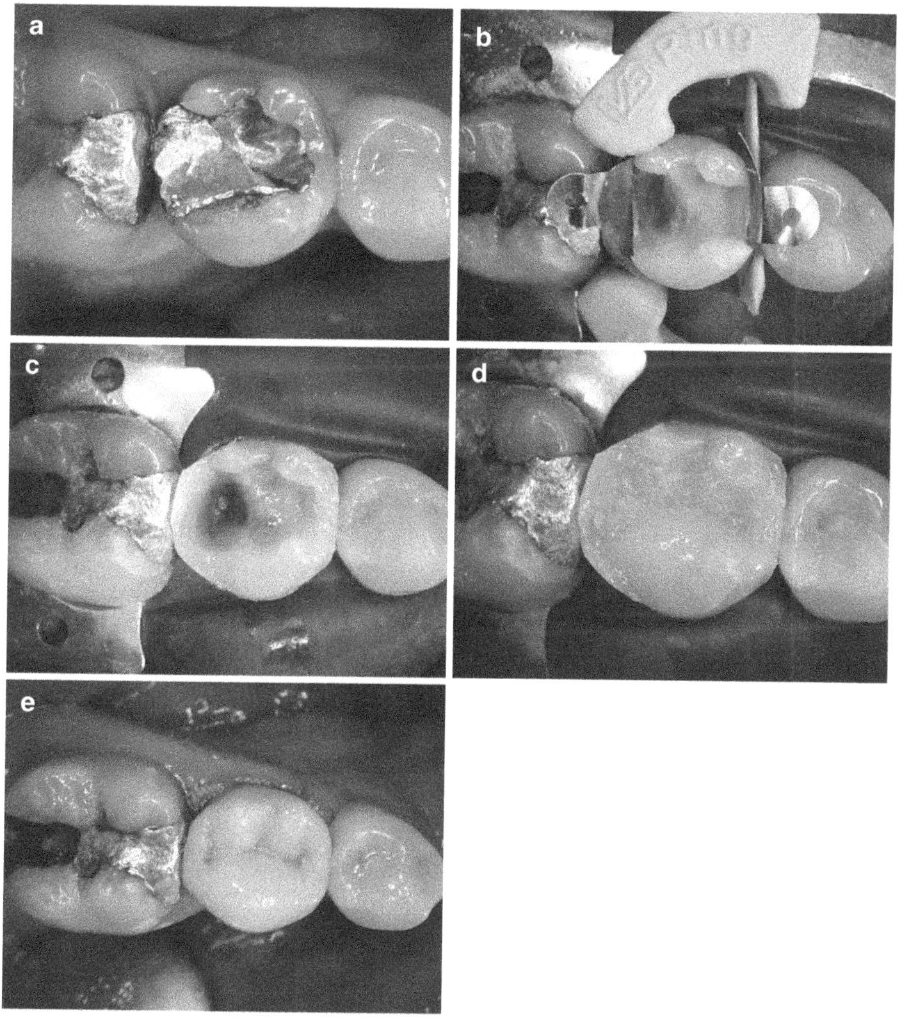

Fig. 7.5 (**a**) Pre-operative view: Clinical view of a defective amalgam restoration in combination with a primary carious lesion at the mesial wall. (**b**) After removal of the old restoration and the carious lesion a dental dam is placed and countered sectional metal matrices in combination with a separation ring. (**c**) Interproximal walls were build-up by PFC according to a centripetal filling technique. (**d**) Missing dentine replaced by a semi-IPN-based bulk short fiber composite base (notice protruding fibers from the SFRC surface). (**e**) Post-operative view: The occlusal part is build-up with hybrid composite and the restoration is finished and adjusted in occlusion

post-curing from the buccal and lingual aspect was performed after matrix removal. Occlusion and articulation were checked and adjusted after removal of the dental dam. The restoration was finished with fine-grit diamond burs (8862 and 862EF; Komet), abrasive discs (OptiDisc; KerrHawe) and strips (Sof-Lex strips; 3 M ESPE) and polished with rubbers (HiLuster; KerrHawe) and brushes (OccluBrush; KerrHawe) (Fig. 7.5e).

7.5.2 Clinical Case: everX Flow

A female patient presented with secondary caries due to a defective Class II amalgam restoration on a lower first molar (FDI #36). This case was treated according to the same principles and protocol as the previous case. The main difference between this and the previous case was the SFRC used, a flowable SFRC (everX Flow) instead of packable SFRC (everX Posterior) for replacing the lost dentine tissue (Fig. 7.6a–f).

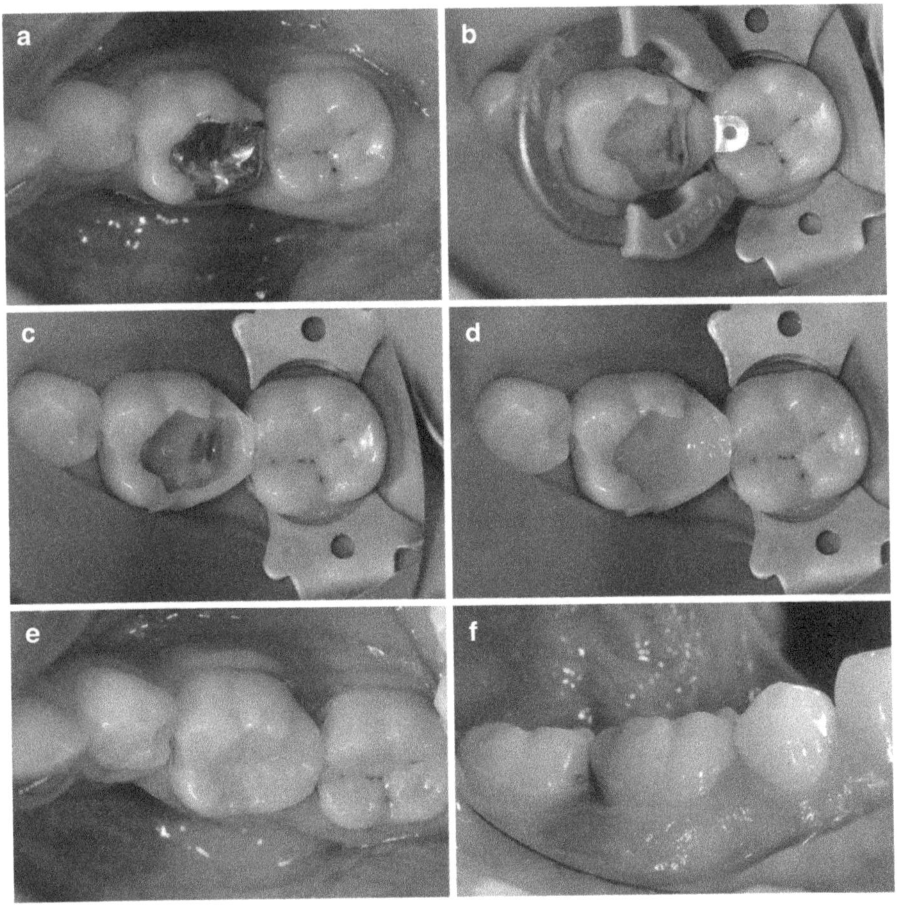

Fig. 7.6 (**a**) Pre-operative view: Clinical view of a defective amalgam restoration and secondary caries on the lower first molar (FDI #36). (**b**) Countered sectional metal matrices in combination with a separation ring is placed in order to rebuild the distal wall, a part of the buccal cusp and the lingual cusp. (**c**) Centripetal filling technique is used to rebuild the missing distal wall and lingual cusp with several portions of enamel-replacing PFC. (**d**) A flowable SFRC (everX Flow) is applied in several increments to replace the missing dentine. (**e, f**) post-operative view: A nanohybrid composite is selected to restore the occlusal part of the tooth

7.6 Conclusion and Future Trends

Many clinical studies for direct and indirect large posterior composite restorations have identified that fracture of the restoration was the most common reason for failure with no significant differences between the two techniques. It is hypothesized that using SFRC substructure could reinforce the composite restoration for use in high stress-bearing areas of the dental arch. The function of the bulk SFRC base is assumed to be based on supporting the superficial conventional PFC and behaving as a crack arrest barrier. In other words, it mimics the natural behavior of enamel and dentine. The present chapter briefly described the structure, properties and benefits of using SFRC in many clinical situations. Within the limitations of this case series of clinical indications, SFRCs are a promising material that give the clinician the opportunity to replace missing tooth tissue in a more biomimetic way. Therefore, SFRCs can be beneficial in large stress-bearing restorations as a dentine-replacing materials, resulting into less fracture-related failures and improving overall longevity of direct and indirect resin composite restorations. Long-term clinical studies are currently in progress to determine the value and usefulness of using bilayered or biomimetic composite restorations made of a high toughness dentine-replacing SFRC and a wear-resistant and highly esthetic PFC as enamel-replacement in high stress-bearing areas.

Future developments in short fiber reinforcement technology are focused now on the optimization of the SFRC CAD/CAM blocks [85–87] and SFRC as 3D printing material, in order to have bilayered composite restorations. Efforts to get even closer in producing a material suitable to replace lost dentine include the investigation of using nanofibers and a compositions and structure closer to an apatite minerals in order to enhance the performance resin composite.

References

1. Manhart J, Kunzelmann KH, Chen HY, Hickel R. Mechanical properties and wear behavior of light-cured packable composite resins. Dent Mater. 2000;16:33–40.
2. Fennis WM, Kuijs RH, Roeters FJ, Creugers NH, Kreulen CM. Randomized control trial of composite cuspal restorations: five-year results. J Dent Res. 2014;93:36–41. https://doi.org/10.1177/0022034513510946.
3. Manhart J, Chen H, Hamm G, Hickel R. Buonocore memorial lecture. Review of the clinical survival of direct and indirect restorations in posterior teeth of the permanent dentition. Oper Dent. 2004;29:481–508.
4. Wilder AD, May KN, Bayne SC, Taylor DF, Leinfelder KF. Seventeen-year clinical study of ultraviolet-cured posterior composite class I and II restorations. J Esthet Dent. 1999;11:135–42.
5. Bowen RL. Properties of a silica-reinforced polymer for dental restorations. J Am Dent Assoc. 1963;66:57–64.
6. Demarco FF, Corrêa MB, Cenci MS, Moraes RR, Opdam NJM. Longevity of posterior composite restorations: not only a matter of materials. Dent Mater. 2012;28:87–101. https://doi.org/10.1016/j.dental.2011.09.003.
7. Brunthaler A, Konig F, Lucas T, Sperr W, Schedle A. Longevity of direct resin composite restorations in posterior teeth. Clin Oral Investig. 2003;7:63–70. https://doi.org/10.1007/s00784-003-0206-7.

8. Bernardo M, Luis H, Martin MD, Leroux BG, Rue T, Leitao J, DeRouen TA. Survival and reasons for failure of amalgam versus composite posterior restorations placed in a randomized clinical trial. J Am Dent Assoc. 2007;138:775–83. https://doi.org/10.14219/jada.archive.2007.0265.
9. Opdam NJ, Bronkhorst EM, Roeters JM, Loomans BA. A retrospective clinical study on longevity of posterior composite and amalgam restorations. Dent Mater. 2007;23:2–8. https://doi.org/10.1016/j.dental.2005.11.036.
10. Van Nieuwenhuysen JP, D'Hoore W, Carvalho J, Qvist V. Long-term evaluation of extensive restorations in permanent teeth. J Dent. 2003;31:395–405.
11. Opdam NJ, Bronkhorst EM, Roeters JM, Loomans BA. Longevity and reasons for failure of sandwich and total-etch posterior composite resin restorations. J Adhes Dent. 2007;9:469–75.
12. Lempel E, Lovász BV, Bihari E, Krajczar K, Jeges S, Toth A, Szalma J. Long-term clinical evaluation of direct resin composite restorations in vital vs. endodontically treated posterior teeth-retrospective study up to 13 years. Dent Mater. 2019;35(9):1308–18. https://doi.org/10.1016/j.dental.2019.06.002.
13. Fennis WM, Kuijs RH, Kreulen C, Roeters FJ, Creugers NH, Burgersdijk RC. A survey of cusp fractures in a population of general dental practices. Int J Prosthodont. 2002;15:559–63.
14. Roulet J-F. Benefits and disadvantages of tooth-coloured alternatives to amalgam. J Dent. 1997;25:459–73. https://doi.org/10.1016/S0300-5712(96)00066-8.
15. Wilder AJ, Bayne S, Ho H. Long-term clinical oerformance of direct posterior composites. Trans Acad Dent Mater. 1996;9:151–69.
16. Xu HH. Dental composite resins containing silica-fused ceramic single-crystalline whiskers with various filler levels. J Dent Res. 1999;78:1304–11.
17. Magne P. Pascal Magne: "it should not be about aesthetics but tooth-conserving dentistry". Interview by Ruth Doherty. Br Dent J. 2012;213:189–91. https://doi.org/10.1038/sj.bdj.2012.769.
18. Keulemans F, Garoushi S, Lassila L. Fillings and core-built ups. In: Vallittu, Özcan, editors. A clinical guide to principles of fiber reinforced composites (FRCs) in dentistry. Cambridge: Woodhead Publishing; 2017.
19. Magne P, Belser U. Understanding the intact tooth and the biomimetic principle. In: Magne P, Belser U, editors. Bonded porcelain restorations in the anterior dentition: a biomimetic approach. Chicago: Quintessence Publishing Co; 2002. p. 23–55.
20. Magne P. Composite resins and bonded porcelain: the postamalgam era? J Calif Dent Assoc. 2006;34:135–47.
21. Garoushi S, Lassila LV, Tezvergil A, Vallittu PK. Load bearing capacity of fiber-reinforced and particulate filler composite resin combination. J Dent. 2006;34:179–84.
22. Garoushi S, Lassila LVJ, Tezvergil A, Vallittu PK. Static and fatigue compression test for particulate filler composite resin with fiber-reinforced composite substructure. Dent Mater. 2007;23:17–23. https://doi.org/10.1016/j.dental.2005.11.041.
23. Garoushi S, Vallittu PK, Lassila LV. Short glass fiber reinforced restorative composite resin with semi-inter penetrating polymer network matrix. Dent Mater. 2007;23:1356–62.
24. Xu HH, Quinn JB, Smith DT, Giuseppetti AA, Eichmiller FC. Effects of different whiskers on the reinforcement of dental resin composites. Dent Mater. 2003;19:359–67. https://doi.org/10.1016/S0109-5641(02)00078-7.
25. Zandinejad AA, Atai M, Pahlevan A. The effect of ceramic and porous fillers on the mechanical properties of experimental dental composites. Dent Mater. 2006;22:382–7. https://doi.org/10.1016/j.dental.2005.04.027.
26. Ferracane JL, Berge HX, Condon JR. In vitro aging of dental composites in water—effect of degree of conversion, filler volume, and filler/matrix coupling. J Biomed Mater Res. 1998;42:465–72.
27. Garoushi S, Sailynoja E, Vallittu PK, Lassila L. Physical properties and depth of cure of a new short fiber reinforced composite. Dent Mater. 2013;29:835–41. https://doi.org/10.1016/j.dental.2013.04.016.

28. Garoushi S, Vallittu PK, Watts DC, Lassila LV. Polymerization shrinkage of experimental short glass fiber-reinforced composite with semi-inter penetrating polymer network matrix. Dent Mater. 2008;24(2):211–5.
29. Garoushi S, Vallittu PK, Lassila L. Mechanical properties and wear of five commercial fiber-reinforced filling materials. Chin J Dent Res. 2017;20(3):137–43.
30. Lassila L, Keulemans F, Vallittu PK, Garoushi S. Characterization of restorative short-fiber reinforced dental composites. Dent Mater J. 2020;39(6):992–9.
31. Garoushi S, Gargoum A, Vallittu PK, Lassila L. Short fiber-reinforced composite restorations: a review of the current literature. J Investig Clin Dent. 2018;9(3):e12330. https://doi.org/10.1111/jicd.12330.
32. Garoushi S, Tanner J, Keulemans F, Le Bell-Rönnlöf AM, Lassila L, Vallittu PK. Fiber reinforcement of endodontically treated teeth: what options do we have? Literature review. Eur J Prosthodont Restor Dent. 2020;28(2):54–63.
33. Vallittu PK. High-aspect ratio fillers: fiber-reinforced composites and their anisotropic properties. Dent Mater. 2014;31:1–7. https://doi.org/10.1016/j.dental.2014.07.009.
34. Lassila L, Garoushi S, Vallittu PK, Säilynoja E. Mechanical properties of fiber reinforced restorative composite with two distinguished fiber length distribution. J Mech Behav Biomed Mater. 2016;60:331–8. https://doi.org/10.1016/j.jmbbm.2016.01.036.
35. Bijelic-Donova J, Garoushi S, Lassila LV, Keulemans F, Vallittu PK. Mechanical and structural characterization of discontinuous fiber-reinforced dental resin composite. J Dent. 2016;52:70–8.
36. Lastumäki TM, Lassila LV, Vallittu PK. The semi-interpenetrating polymer network matrix of fiber-reinforced composite and its effect on the surface adhesive properties. J Mater Sci Mater Med. 2003;14:803–9.
37. Fagundes TC, Barata TJ, Carvalho CA, Franco EB, van Dijken JW, Navarro MF. Clinical evaluation of two packable posterior composites: a five-year follow-up. J Am Dent Assoc. 2009;140:447–54. https://doi.org/10.14219/jada.archive.2009.0194. 140/4/447[pii]
38. van Dijken JW, Sunnegardh-Gronberg K. Fiber-reinforced packable resin composites in class II cavities. J Dent. 2006;34:763–9.
39. Heintze SD, Ilie N, Hickel R, Reis A, Loguercio A, Rousson V. Laboratory mechanical parameters of composite resins and their relation to fractures and wear in clinical trials-a systematic review. Dent Mater. 2017;33:101–14.
40. Lassila L, Säilynoja E, Prinssi R, Vallittu P, Garoushi S. Characterization of a new fiber-reinforced flowable composite. Odontology. 2019;107(3):342–52.
41. Garoushi S, Vallittu P, Lassila L. Mechanical properties and radiopacity of flowable fiber-reinforced composite. Dent Mater J. 2019;38(2):196–202.
42. Garoushi S, Vallittu PK, Lassila LV. Fracture toughness, compressive strength and load-bearing capacity of short glass fiber-reinforced composite resin. Chin J Dent Res. 2011;14:15–9.
43. Petersen RC. Discontinuous fiber-reinforced composites above critical length. J Dent Res. 2005;84:365–70.
44. Tiu J, Belli R, Lohbauer U. R-curve behavior of a short-fiber reinforced resin composite after water storage. J Mech Behav Biomed Mater. 2020;104:103674.
45. Tiu J, Belli R, Lohbauer U. Rising R-curves in particulate/fiber-reinforced resin composite layered systems. J Mech Behav Biomed Mater. 2020;103:103537.
46. Abouelleil H, Pradelle N, Villat C, Colon P, Grosgogeat B. Comparison of mechanical properties of a new fiber reinforced composite and bulk filling composites. Restor Dent Endod. 2015;7658:1–8.
47. Lassila L, Keulemans F, Säilynoja E, Vallittu PK, Garoushi S. Mechanical properties and fracture behavior of flowable fiber reinforced composite restorations. Dent Mater. 2018;34(4):598–606.
48. Ilie N, Hickel R, Valceanu AS, Huth KC. Fracture toughness of dental restorative materials. Clin Oral Investig. 2012;16:489–98. https://doi.org/10.1007/s00784-011-0525-z.

49. Tsujimoto A, Barkmeier WW, Takamizawa T, Watanabe H, Johnson WW, Latta MA, Miyazaki M. Relationship between mechanical properties and bond durability of short fiber-reinforced resin composite with universal adhesive. Eur J Oral Sci. 2016;124:480–9.
50. Omran TA, Garoushi S, Abdulmajeed AA, Lassila LV, Vallittu PK. Influence of increment thickness on dentin bond strength and light transmission of composite base materials. Clin Oral Investig. 2017;21(5):1717–24.
51. Garoushi S, Vallittu P, Shinya A, Lassila L. Influence of increment thickness on light transmission, degree of conversion and micro hardness of bulk fill composites. Odontology. 2015;104(3):291–7. https://doi.org/10.1007/s10266-015-0227-0.
52. Miletic V, Pongprueksa P, De., Munck, J., Brooks, N.R., Van., Meerbeek, B. Curing characteristics of flowable and sculptable bulk-fill composites. Clin Oral Investig. 2017;21(4): 1201–12.
53. Lassila L, Säilynoja E, Prinssi R, Vallittu PK, Garoushi S. The effect of polishing protocol on surface gloss of different restorative resin composites. Biomater Investig Dent. 2020;7:1–8.
54. Moorthy A, Hogg CH, Dowling AH, Grufferty BF, Benetti AR, Fleming GJP. Cuspal deflection and microleakage in premolar teeth restored with bulk-fill flowable resin-based composite base materials. J Dent. 2012;40:500–5. https://doi.org/10.1016/j.jdent.2012.02.015.
55. Garoushi S, Tanner J, Vallittu P, Lassila L. Preliminary clinical evaluation of short fiber-reinforced composite resin in posterior teeth: 12-months report. Open Dent J. 2012;6:41–5. https://doi.org/10.2174/1874210601206010041TODENTJ-6-41.
56. Tanner J, Tolvanen M, Garoushi S, Säilynoja E. Clinical evaluation of fiber-reinforced composite restorations in posterior teeth-results of 2.5 year follow-up. Open Dent J. 2018;12: 476–85.
57. ElAziz RH, Mohammed MM, Gomaa HAF. Clinical performance of short-fiber-reinforced resin composite restorations vs resin composite onlay restorations in complex cavities of molars (randomized clinical trial). J Contemp Dent Pract. 2020;21(3):296–303.
58. Garoushi S, Vallittu PK, Lassila LV. Use of short fiber-reinforced composite with semi-interpenetrating polymer network matrix in fixed partial dentures. J Dent. 2007;35: 403–8.
59. Garoushi SK, Lassila LV, Vallittu PK. Fiber-reinforced composite substructure: load-bearing capacity of an onlay restoration. Acta Odontol Scand. 2006;64:281–5.
60. Garoushi S, Vallittu PK, Lassila LV. Fracture resistance of short, randomly oriented, glass fiber-reinforced composite premolar crowns. Acta Biomater. 2007;3:779–84.
61. Garoushi S, Vallittu PK, Lassila LV. Direct restoration of severely damaged incisors using short fiber-reinforced composite resin. J Dent. 2007;35:731–6.
62. Garoushi SK, Hatem M, Lassila LVJ, Vallittu PK. The effect of short fiber composite base on microleakage and load-bearing capacity of posterior restorations. Acta Biomater Odontol Scand. 2015;1:6–12. https://doi.org/10.3109/23337931.2015.1017576.
63. Keulemans F, Palav P, Aboushelib MMN, van Dalen A, Kleverlaan CJ, Feilzer AJ. Fracture strength and fatigue resistance of dental resin-based composites. Dent Mater. 2009;25:1433–41. https://doi.org/10.1016/j.dental.2009.06.013.
64. Fráter M, Forster A, Keresztúri M, Braunitzer G, Nagy K. In vitro fracture resistance of molar teeth restored with a short fiber-reinforced composite material. J Dent. 2014;42:1143–50. https://doi.org/10.1016/j.jdent.2014.05.004.
65. Bijelic J, Garoushi S, Vallittu PK, Lassila LV. Short fiber reinforced composite in restoring severely damaged incisors. Acta Odontol Scand. 2013;71:1221–31. https://doi.org/10.3109/00016357.2012.757640.
66. Sáry T, Garoushi S, Braunitzer G, Alleman D, Volom A, Fráter M. Fracture behaviour of MOD restorations reinforced by various fiber-reinforced techniques—an in vitro study. J Mech Behav Biomed Mater. 2019;98:348–56. [published correction appears in J Mech Behav Biomed Mater. 2020 Feb;102:103505]. https://doi.org/10.1016/j.jmbbm.2019.07.006.
67. Szabó B, Garoushi S, Braunitzer G, Szabó PB, Baráth Z, Fráter M. Fracture behavior of root-amputated teeth at different amount of periodontal support—a preliminary in vitro

study. BMC Oral Health. 2019;19(1):261. Published 2019 Nov 27. https://doi.org/10.1186/s12903-019-0958-3.
68. Garoushi S, Mangoush E, Vallittu PK, Lassila L. Short fiber reinforced composite: a new alternative for direct onlay restorations. Open Dent J. 2013;7:181–5. Published 2013 Dec 30. https://doi.org/10.2174/1874210601307010181.
69. Ozsevik AS, Yildirim C, Aydin U, Culha E, Surmelioglu D. Effect of fiber-reinforced composite on the fracture resistance of endodontically treated teeth. Aust Endod J. 2015;42(2):82–7. http://www.ncbi.nlm.nih.gov/pubmed/26611674. Accessed 5 Nov 16.
70. Fráter M, Sáry T, Néma V, Braunitzer G, Vallittu PK, Lassila L, Garoushi S. Fatigue failure load of immature anterior teeth: influence of different fiber post-core systems. Odontology. 2020;10:222–30. https://doi.org/10.1007/s10266-020-00522-y.
71. Lassila L, Oksanen V, Fráter M, Vallittu PK, Garoushi S. The influence of resin composite with high fiber aspect ratio on fracture resistance of severely damaged bovine incisors. Dent Mater J. 2020;39(3):381–8. https://doi.org/10.4012/dmj.2019-051.
72. Fráter M, Lassila L, Braunitzer G, Vallittu PK, Garoushi S. Fracture resistance and marginal gap formation of post-core restorations: influence of different fiber-reinforced composites. Clin Oral Investig. 2020;24(1):265–76.
73. Fráter M, Sáry T, Jókai B, Braunitzer G, Säilynoja E, Vallittu PK, Lassila L, Garoushi S. Fatigue behavior of endodontically treated premolars restored with different fiber-reinforced designs. Dent Mater. 2021;37(3):391–402.
74. Keulemans F, Van Dalen A, Kleverlaan CJ, Feilzer AJ. Static and dynamic failure load of fiber-reinforced composite and particulate filler composite cantilever resin-bonded fixed dental prostheses. J Adhes Dent. 2010;12:207–14. https://doi.org/10.3290/j.jad.a17653.
75. Keulemans F, De Jager N, Kleverlaan CJ, Feilzer AJ. Influence of retainer design on two-unit cantilever resin-bonded glass fiber reinforced composite fixed dental prostheses: an in vitro and finite element analysis study. J Adhes Dent. 2008;10:355–64.
76. Bijelic-Donova J, Garoushi S, Vallittu PK, Lassila LVJ. Mechanical properties, fracture resistance, and fatigue limits of short fiber reinforced dental composite resin. J Prosthet Dent. 2016;115:95–102. https://doi.org/10.1016/j.prosdent.2015.07.012.
77. Lassila L, Säilynoja E, Prinssi R, Vallittu PK, Garoushi S. Fracture behavior of bi-structure fiber-reinforced composite restorations. J Mech Behav Biomed Mater. 2020;101:103444. https://doi.org/10.1016/j.jmbbm.2019.103444.
78. Nagata K, Garoushi SK, Vallittu PK, Wakabayashi N, Takahashi H, Lassila LVJ. Fracture behavior of single-structure fiber-reinforced composite restorations. Acta Biomater Odontol Scand. 2016;2(1):118–24. Published 2016 Sep 5. https://doi.org/10.1080/23337931.2016.1224670.
79. Bijelic-Donova J, Keulemans F, Vallittu PK, Lassila LVJ. Direct bilayered biomimetic composite restoration: the effect of a cusp-supporting short fiber-reinforced base design on the chewing fracture resistance and failure mode of molars with or without endodontic treatment. J Mech Behav Biomed Mater. 2020;103:103554.
80. Lassila L, Säilynoja E, Prinssi R, Vallittu P, Garoushi S. Bilayered composite restoration: the effect of layer thickness on fracture behavior. Biomater Investig Dent. 2020;7(1):80–5.
81. Garoushi S, Sungur S, Boz Y, Ozkan P, Vallittu PK, Uctasli S, Lassila L. Influence of short-fiber composite base on fracture behavior of direct and indirect restorations. Clin Oral Investig. 2021;25(7):4543–52.
82. Omran TA, Garoushi S, Lassila L, Shinya A, Vallittu PK. Bonding interface affects the load-bearing capacity of bilayered composites. Dent Mater J. 2019;38(6):1002–11. https://doi.org/10.4012/dmj.2018-304.
83. Omran TA, Garoushi S, Lassila LV, Vallittu PK. Effect of interface surface design on the fracture behavior of bilayered composites. Eur J Oral Sci. 2019;127(3):276–84. https://doi.org/10.1111/eos.12617.
84. Imbeni V, Kruzic JJ, Marshall GW, Marshall SJ, Ritchie RO. The dentin-enamel junction and the fracture of human teeth. Nat Mater. 2005;4:229–32.

85. Mangoush E, Garoushi S, Vallittu PK, Lassila L. Influence of short fiber- reinforced composites on fracture resistance of single-structure restorations. Eur J Prosthodont Restor Dent. 2020;28(4):189–98.
86. Mangoush E, Lassila L, Vallittu PK, Garoushi S. Microstructure and surface characteristics of short-FIBER reinforced CAD/CAM composite blocks. Eur J Prosthodont Restor Dent. 2021;29(3).
87. Mangoush E, Lassila L, Vallittu PK, Garoushi S. Shear-bond strength and optical properties of short fiber-reinforced CAD/CAM composite blocks. Eur J Oral Sci. 2021;129(5):e12815.

Guidelines for Achieving Aesthetic Posterior Restorations Using BFCs

8

Joseph Sabbagh, Robert McConnell, and Alessandro Vichi

8.1 Introduction

In 2014 Christopher Ho (in Principles and Practice of Esthetic Dentistry) [1] wrote that aesthetic dentistry is a marriage between the 'art and science of dentistry'. He goes on to explain that the clinician should possess an intimate knowledge of the different aesthetic materials available, and their clinical indications, application, and limitations in practice. The clinician should have or acquire the skills to carry out a functional and aesthetic restoration.

This is especially true when one is restoring complex posterior cavities with a material whose physical properties include polymerization shrinkage, moisture sensitivity, etc. Patients are now more demanding and expect aesthetic posterior restorations. The clinician should include in their assessment and choice of posterior filling material any unmet or possibly unrealistic, expectations from their patients.

These and other elements will be outlined to provide and maintain successful aesthetic posterior restorations for our patients.

The shift from amalgam to composite for restoring larger cavities in the posterior dentition highlighted the many undesirable properties of resin-based materials. Placing resin composite in posterior teeth was technically more difficult and

J. Sabbagh (✉)
Department of Restorative and Aesthetic Dentistry and Endodontics, Faculty of Dental Medicine, Lebanese University, Beirut, Lebanon
e-mail: josephsabbagh@ul.edu.lb

R. McConnell
Restorative Dentistry, University Dental School and Hospital, University College Cork, Cork, Ireland
e-mail: r.mcconnell@ucc.ie

A. Vichi
Dental Academy, University of Portsmouth, Portsmouth, UK
e-mail: alessandro.vichi@port.ac.uk

J. Sabbagh, R. McConnell (eds.), *Bulk Fill Resin Composites in Dentistry*,
https://doi.org/10.1007/978-3-031-16388-3_8

unpredictable. Unlike amalgam, resin materials tended to adhere to instruments, often resulting in the inclusion of voids within the restoration itself especially at the bottom of the cavity. Polymerization shrinkage as well as other factors such as matrix placement and adaptation made achieving a tight contact with the adjacent tooth a challenge.

To address these and other clinical challenges, packable resin composite materials were first introduced. These materials had improved mechanical properties and it was thought would make achieving a tight contact point easier. However, it was soon discovered that these materials were not superior to any universal hybrid composites [2, 3] and did not help to improve the creation of a tight contact point [4].

The placement of a thin layer of flowable composite on the cavity floor when using packable materials was advised to improve the adaptation of the material to the floor of the cavity. However, several studies noted that the use of flowable resin composite as an intermediate material did not reduce microleakage or improve gingival margin adaptation [5, 6].

In 2020, Ferracane et al. [7] investigated the best strategy for the placement of resin composites into a class II cavity and found that in vitro and clinical evidence available did not support any specific method or material type for achieving optimal performance. In this publication the authors suggested that the most important factor for achieving success was most likely to be the careful and proper placement of the material by the operator followed by an appropriate light curing technique.

8.2 Bulk Filling Materials

Bulk fill resin composites were developed to offer the dentist a faster filling and curing composites for restoring posterior cavities, using a layer of up to 4 mm. Since many dentists worldwide were trained to restore posterior teeth using amalgam and do not use rubber dam for the placement of posterior restorations [8], this material and technique has gained popularity for achieving predictable posterior composite restorations. Linking their use with self-etch adhesive system, bulk filling restorative material offers the dentist a predictable high-quality restoration in a shorter time as well as several other clinical advantages [9, 10].

These materials are especially useful when restoring posterior cavities where procedural time is of concern. This may include children and anxious patients where the length of treatment time is ideally kept short.

They offer an aesthetic tooth-coloured restorative material which is less technique sensitive to conventional composites. There is evidence of better adaptation of the material to the walls of the cavity with fewer voids all leading to less microleakage of the restoration [11, 12].

A method to increase the degree of polymerization of bulk fill materials is to increase their translucency [13]. This will allow a better diffusion of the light with increased polymerization depth and extent [11, 14, 15]. It is a well-known effect that when the translucency increase, composite materials tend to have a lower value (lightness or brightness). In other words, the restoration becomes greyish. This is a commonly observed effect in bulk restorative materials, particularly with low viscosity bulk fill materials. This characteristic may pose problems when using a layering technique. As an example, if the well-known centripetal build-up technique [16] is practiced, the first layer applied is in the interproximal box. This will improve the C-factor and transform a class II cavity into a class I cavity. If a bulk fill translucent material is used, there is the risk that the interproximal area might have an unesthetic greyish appearance. This is particularly evident when the adjacent tooth is a porcelain fused to metal restoration. In this case, it would be preferable to limit occlusally the resin composite material (leaving room for a final layer) and filling the remaining "Class I" cavity with a low viscosity bulk fill material limiting the occlusal extension. Finally (occlusal) place a high-viscosity bulk fill or a traditional hybrid material.

Alternatively, to switch from the centripetal build-up technique to a horizontal layering [12, 17], placing the low viscosity material horizontally in 1–2 layers and then placing a high-viscosity bulk fill (or a hybrid) as the final occlusal layer. This way of layering is probably easier and faster, but, depending on the position of the contact point, the interproximal wall may be made with a low viscosity bulk fill which is not ideal.

Resin composites can mimic the optical properties of the natural tooth. Bulk fill materials offer the ability for a single increment fill technique. Using new low-stress monomers, highly reactive photo-initiators, and different types of nanosized fillers, they are ideal for restoring posterior teeth [14].

8.3 Finishing and Polishing

Another important parameter controlling the aesthetics of composite restorations is finishing and polishing. Currently there are no specific finishing and polishing procedure proposed for bulk fill materials so finishing and polishing systems for conventional microhybrid resin composites are recommended. There have been few studies looking at finishing and polishing of these materials. Differences in filler type and size between high-viscosity bulk fill and traditional nanohybrid resin composites, as well as among the various high-viscosity bulk fill resin composites available are expected to affect their polishability.

As for all resin composite restorations polishability is a critical property as surface characteristics such as roughness and gloss play an important role in determining the clinical outcomes of the restorations. Inadequately finished and polished surfaces are more prone to wear and plaque accumulation, exposing the restored tooth to a higher risk of staining, secondary caries, and gingival irritation [18, 19] possibly compromising the clinical success [20–22]. Furthermore, it is well known that restorations with smooth surfaces are more comfortable, more aesthetically pleasing and better accepted by patients [23, 24].

Several finishing and polishing systems for resin composite restorations is currently available and described in the literature [25–28]. While the effects of finishing and polishing on roughness and gloss of “conventional” hybrid and nanohybrid resin composites have been largely investigated [12, 15, 16]. little evidence has so far been collected about the effects of finishing and polishing procedures on bulk fill materials. Some studies have reported them to be 2–7 times rougher than nano-filled resin composites [29, 30].

Roughness and gloss are clinically relevant characteristics of restorative materials. Roughness is related to irregularities, and it is usually evaluated as roughness average (Ra), which is defined as the mean arithmetical value of all the absolute distances of the profile inside of the measuring length [31]. Gloss is an attribute of visual appearance that involves specular reflection from a surface, it is responsible for lustrous or mirror-like appearance [32, 33], and it is measured in terms of gloss units (GU). Gloss is influenced by how light is reflected from the surface as well as by the refractive indices of resin matrix and filler [34]. Gloss was also found to be affected by filler size and filler-matrix homogeneity, with the observation that the lower the filler-matrix homogeneity, the lower the light reflectivity [35]. There is an inverse linear relationship between gloss and roughness [36].

The purpose of a finishing/polishing procedure is to provide enamel-like surfaces, ideally the final composite roughness should be like enamel-to-enamel contact in occlusal areas (0.64 μm) [37]. Paolone et al. [29] performed a study in which several finishing and polishing system were investigated. In their study, roughness ranged from 0.11 μm to 0.69 μm and all polishing systems provided clinically acceptable results, even if statistically significant differences emerged among the materials and the finishing systems. The authors concluded that their findings could be related to the characteristics of the filler and to the filler size.

The finishing/polishing procedures are also aimed at providing the restoration surface with an enamel-like gloss. There is little agreement in the literature of the desired gloss unit (GU) with Mormann et al. [38] reporting 53 GU to be the reference value for the gloss of polished enamel, while Barucci-Pfister et al. [39] stated that the final gloss of a RC should be within the range of 40–53 GU. Furthermore, no agreement has yet been reached in the literature on the geometry of viewing for gloss measurements, and the lack of uniformity in the experimental set-up among different studies does not allow for a direct comparison of the published results. Some authors reported that a 20° angle enables a better differentiation than a 60° angle [40] while others reported the 45° angle as the best to detect between-material differences [32]. Cook and Thomas [41] using a 60° measurement angle classified as “poor” a finish below 60 GU, as “acceptable” a 60–70 GU finish, and as “excellent” a finish above 80 GU.

Paolone et al. [29] reported that while bulk fill materials enable a time-saving filling technique, there is still no consensus as to whether they also allow a simplified time-saving finishing/polishing procedure. They also reported that 1-, 2-, and 3-steps silicon points differed significantly from a 2-step wheel system and that irrespective of the number of steps, the chemical composition of the polishing points could affect the outcome of the procedure. Many of the polishing systems available contain silicon carbide or aluminium. It should be considered that as of today the polishing system used on some bulk fill available on the market provided clinical acceptable results in terms of roughness, while poor results were achieved in terms of gloss. The indication coming from literature suggested that there is a need to develop a polishing system dedicated to high-viscosity bulk fill resin composite.

8.4 Clinical Application of Bulk Fill Composites

When deciding to restore a posterior cavity with resin composite, several features of the cavity will guide the dentist in their selecting of the most appropriate material including the depth of the cavity; the remaining tooth structure; and the location. Bulk fill resin composites are indicated for medium to deep posterior cavities in permanent teeth (Class I and II). They can also be used to build-up and fill access cavities of root treated teeth, with or without fibre posts, prior to crown placement.

For cavities less than 4 mm depth, one layer of composite material is sufficient to restore the cavity, while for deeper cavities, two to three layers may be required.

Figure 8.1 represents the different clinical indications for bulk fill resin composites.

The following clinical cases represent five different subgroups of bulk fill resin composites.

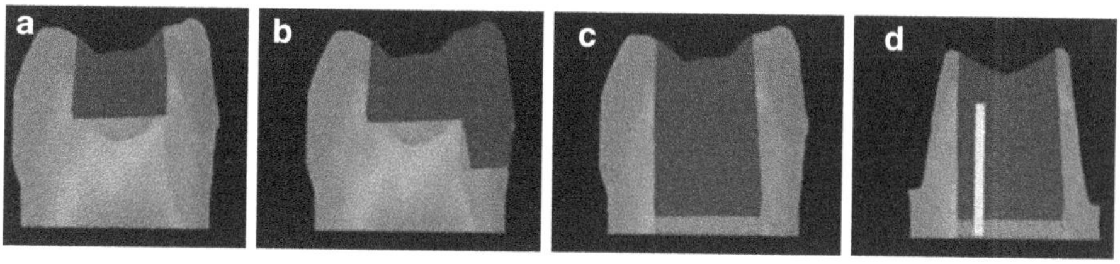

Fig. 8.1 Different indications of bulk fill materials. (**a**) Class I, (**b**) Class II, (**c**) Restoration of Access cavity, (**d**) Tooth build-up using bulk fill and fibre post. (Reprinted from Biomatériaux Cliniques • Vol. 2 - n° 1 mars 2017)

Case 8.1: Use of Flowable Bulk Base Resin Composite, X-Tra Base (Voco)
A young 11-year-old patient presents with sensitivity on tooth number 16 (upper right first molar). Clinical and radiographic examination confirm the presence of a deep caries lesion (Fig. 8.2). Following the administration of local anaesthesia, the cavity was prepared using a pear-shaped diamond bur while the caries was removed using a round metallic bur mounted on a blue contra-angle handpiece. Rubber dam was placed and 37% orthophosphoric etchant was selectively applied to the enamel surfaces (Fig. 8.3).

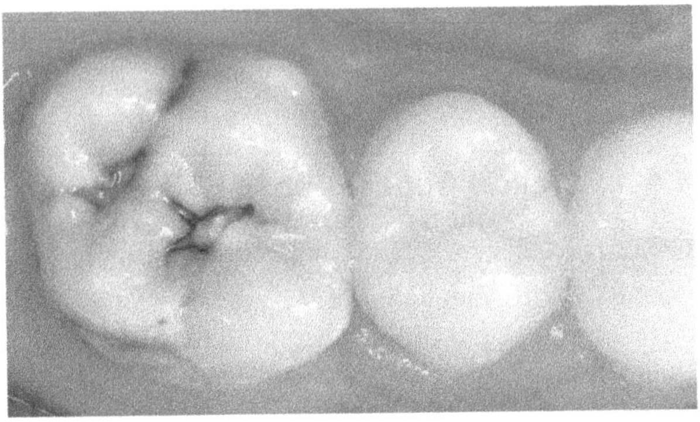

Fig. 8.2 Preoperative view of tooth 16 showing primary caries

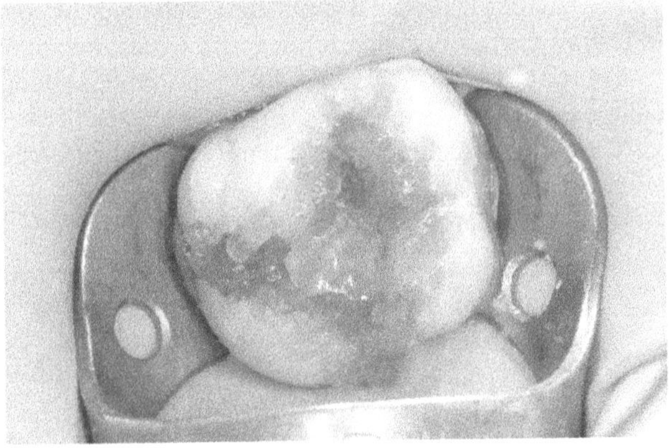

Fig. 8.3 Selective application of 37% phosphoric acid on enamel during 20 s

After rinsing and drying of the cavity, a self-etch adhesive (Futura Bond U, Voco) was applied using a microbrush on the cavity walls, and light cured for 20 s (Fig. 8.4). A bulk fill flowable composite (X-tra Base, shade U, Voco) was injected into the class I cavity up to 1 mm from the occlusal surface and light cured for 40 s (Figs. 8.5, 8.6, and 8.7). The last occlusal millimetre was filled using the Amaris TU (Voco), a nanohybrid composite which gives better wear resistance of the restoration (Fig. 8.8). Figure 8.9 shows the final restoration after finishing and polishing using fine diamond burs and silicone abrasive points.

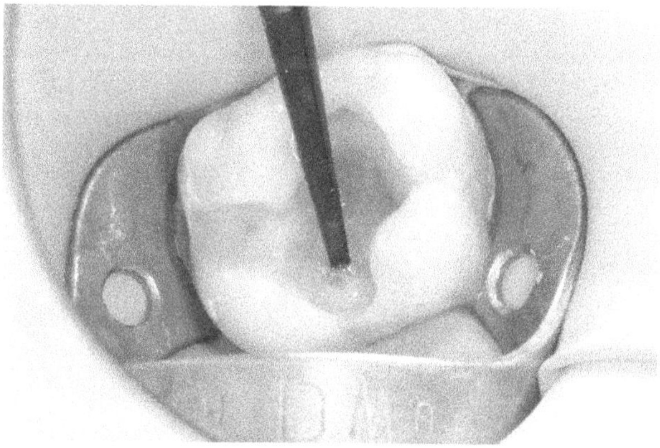

Fig. 8.4 Application of Futura Bond U using a microbrush with scrubbing motion

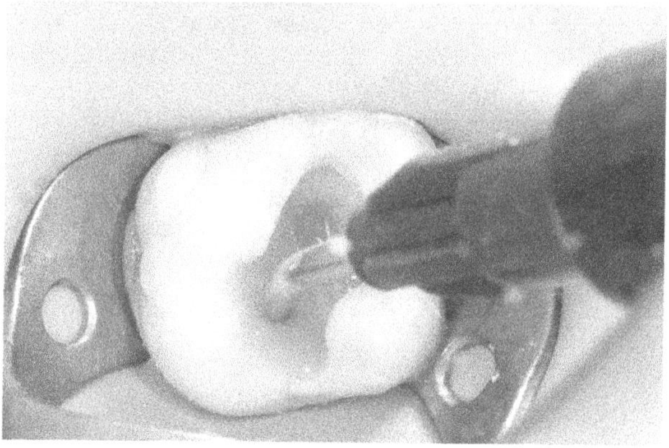

Fig. 8.5 Injection of bulk fill flowable composite (X-tra Base, shade U, Voco) into the class I cavity

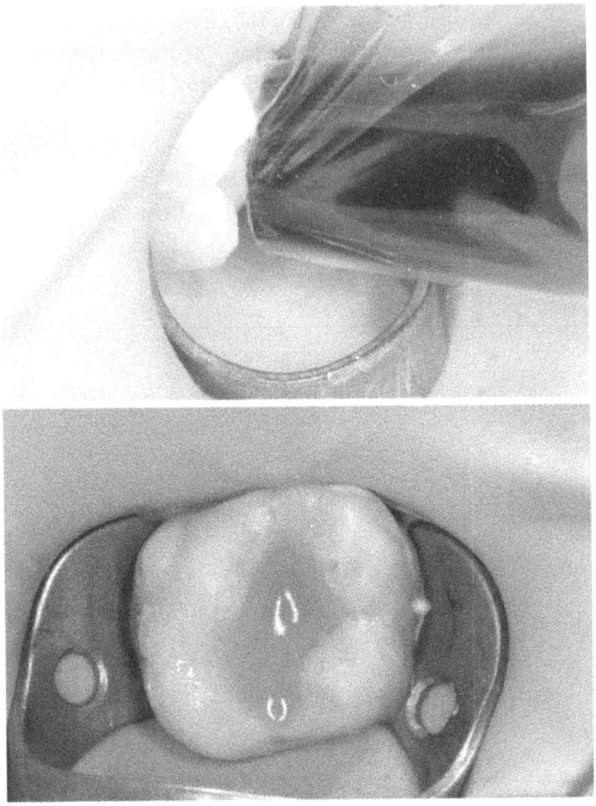

Figs. 8.6 and 8.7 Polymerization of the bulk composite using a LED during 40 s

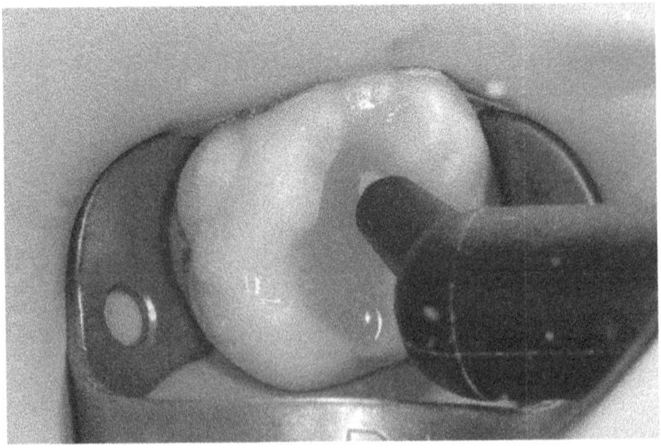

Fig. 8.8 Placement of a layer of Amaris TU for occlusal coverage

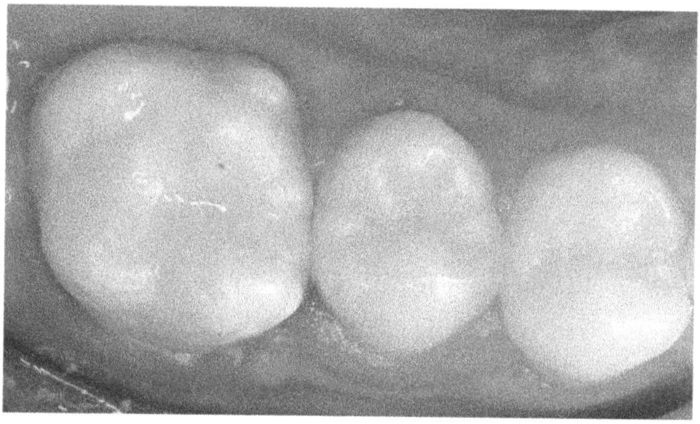

Fig. 8.9 Postoperative view of the final restoration, after finishing and polishing

Case 8.2: Use of Flowable Fibre Based Bulk Fill Resin Composite, EverX-Flow (GC, Tokyo-Japan)

A 35-year-old patient had a root canal treatment on the first upper left molar following pulp necrosis. The proximal contours of the tooth were sound and resistant and so it was decided to fill the access cavity using bulk fill technique (Fig. 8.10). The EverX Flowable resin composite, containing glass fibres, was chosen to restore the tooth. The fibres are believed to reinforce the resin composite by preventing crack propagation [42, 43].

After rubber dam placement, the temporary restoration was removed using a diamond bur under copious water irrigation (Fig. 8.11). A round metallic bur was used to clean the walls of the cavity and remove any residual caries and debris.

After 20 s of etching using 37% phosphoric acid, a universal adhesive system was applied in the cavity, G-Premio (GC, Tokyo-Japan) (Figs. 8.12 and 8.13) and polymerized for 20 s.

EverX Flow was injected in the cavity in a 4 mm layer (Figs. 8.14 and 8.15), and the occlusal 1.5 mm was filled using microhybrid universal Geanial Ac'Hord (GC, Tokyo-Japan) shade A2 (Figs. 8.16 and 8.17). The occlusion was checked using articulating paper, and fine diamond burs were used to remove any prematurity or excess contact. The composite was polished using silicone polishing points, followed by diamond paste resulting in a better polish and lustre (Fig. 8.18).

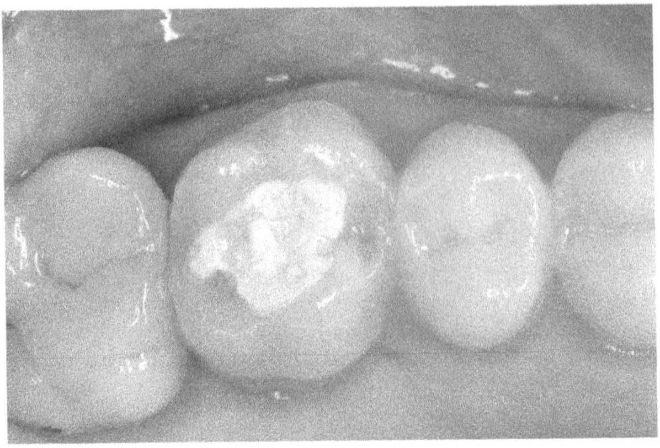

Fig. 8.10 Preoperative view of the access cavity filled with temporary cement

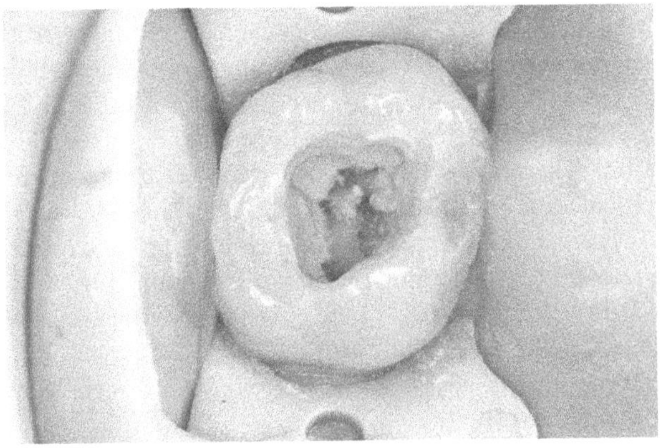

Fig. 8.11 Cavity after removal of the temporary restoration and rubber dam isolation

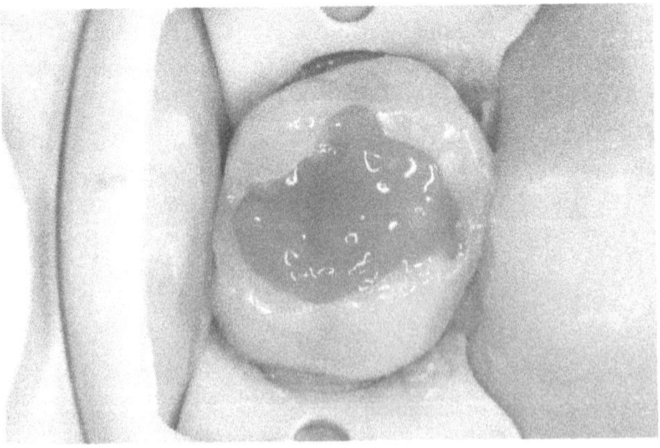

Fig. 8.12 Application of 37% phosphoric acid on enamel during 20 s

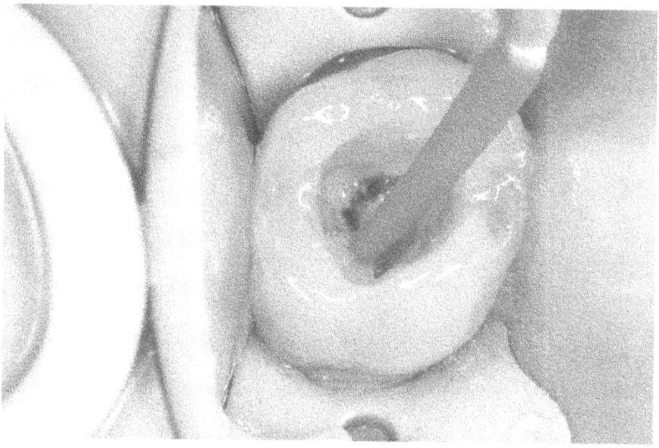

Fig. 8.13 Application of the G-Premio Universal adhesive on the cavity walls

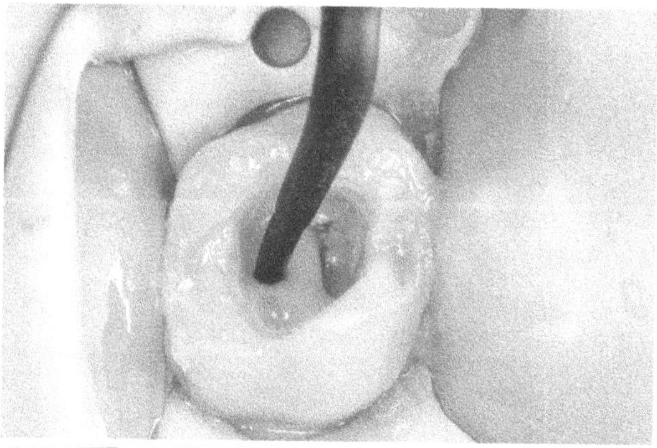

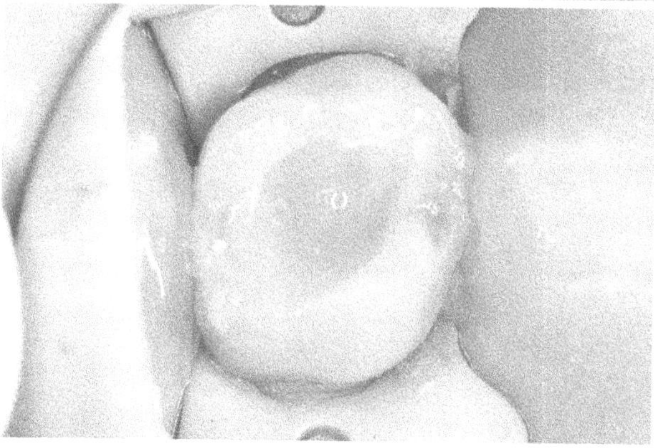

Figs. 8.14 and 8.15 Injection of EverX Flow, fibre based bulk fill composite in the cavity

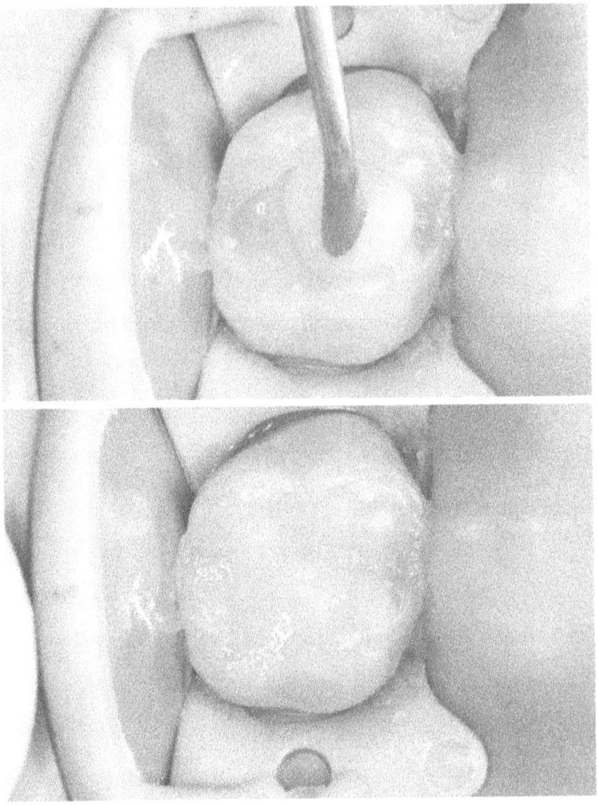

Figs. 8.16 and 8.17 A layer of Geanial Ac'Hord is used on the occlusal surface

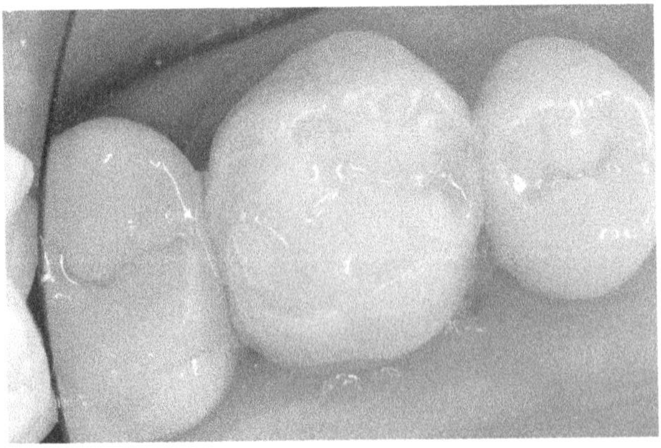

Fig. 8.18 Final composite restoration after finishing and polishing

Case 8.3: Use of Sonically Activated Bulk Fill Resin Composite, Sonicfill 2 (Kavo-Kerr)

A 44-year-old patient presents for a routine check-up, and upon clinical and radiographic examination, two secondary caries lesions were detected on the two upper right molars (teeth 16 and 17) (Fig. 8.19).

Following local anaesthesia, cavities were prepared under copious water irrigation. Caries was removed using a round carbide bur on a contra-angle handpiece. The working field was isolated using a preformed 3D rubber dam, Optidam (Kerr-Kavo) fixed with a Softclamp. Additional ligatures were applied around the teeth, using dental floss, to improve the isolation, and prevent leakage (Fig. 8.20).

A Medium size, Metafix matrix (Kerr-Kavo), was applied on the first tooth (Fig. 8.21) and stabilized with two wooden wedges placed mesially and distally.

OptiBond XTR (Kerr-Kavo), a sixth generation, two component self-adhesive system, was used according to the manufacturer's instructions. The self-etch primer was applied using a microbrush, scrubbed for 20 s and then gently air dried. The bonding resin was then brushed actively for 15 s to allow better penetration in the dentine tubules, air thinned for 5 s and polymerized for 20 s using a LED Demi Ultra curing light (Figs. 8.22, 8.23, 8.24, and 8.25).

Fig. 8.19 Preoperative view of the restorations

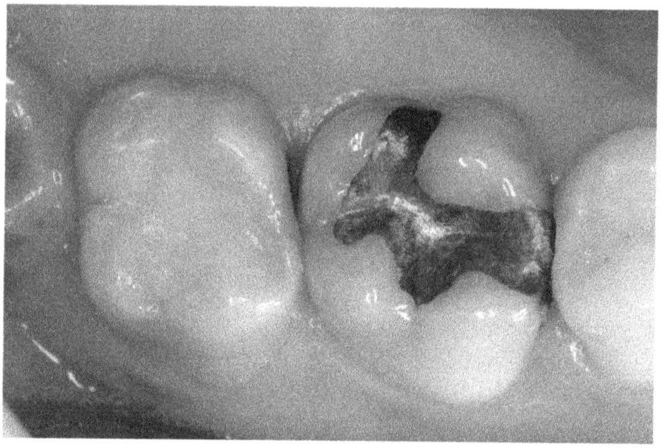

Fig. 8.20 Prepared cavities isolated using OptiDam and Softclamp

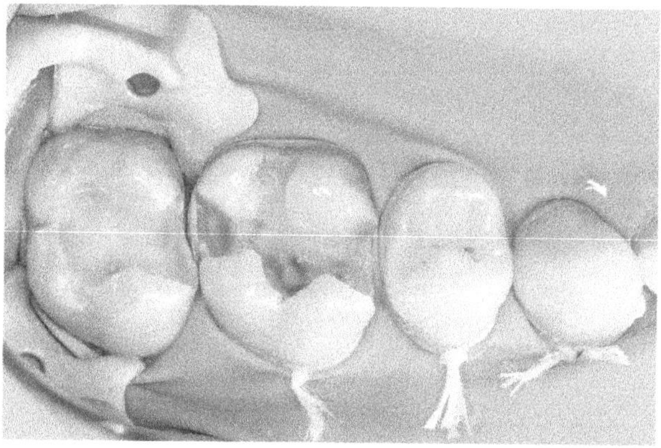

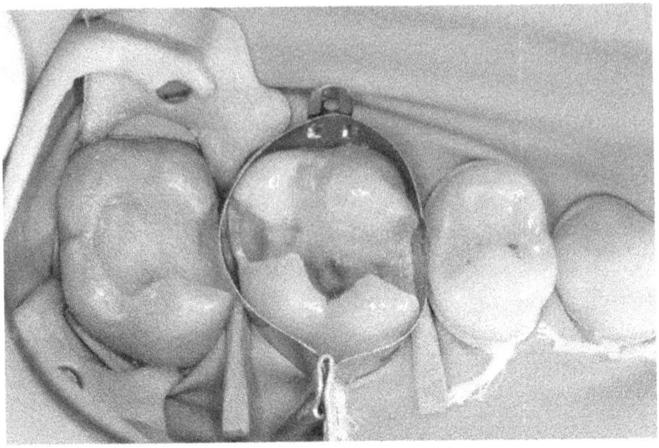

Fig. 8.21 Metafix and woodwedges placement on tooth 16

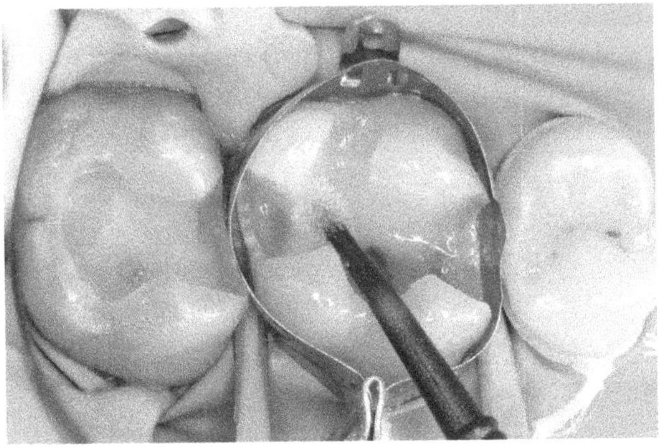

Fig. 8.22 Application of Optibond XTR prime with scrubbing motion

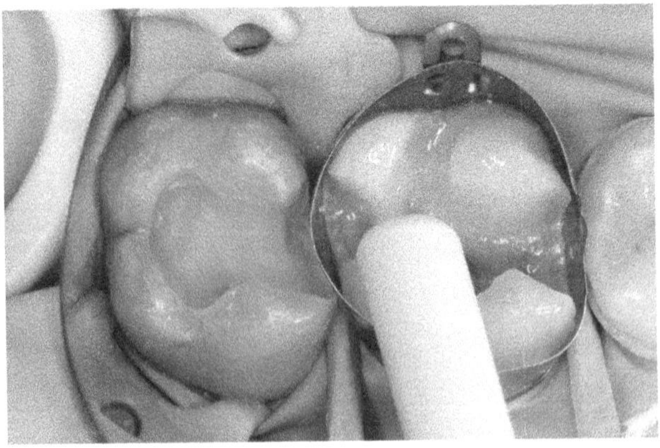

Fig. 8.23 Gentle air dry of the primer

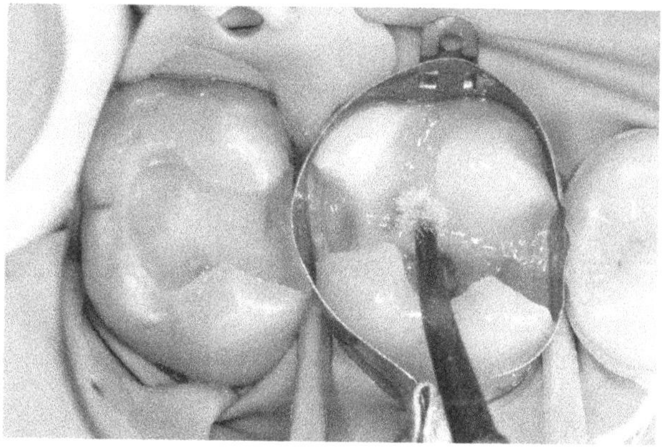

Fig. 8.24 Light brushing of the Optibond XTR bonding agent using a microbrush

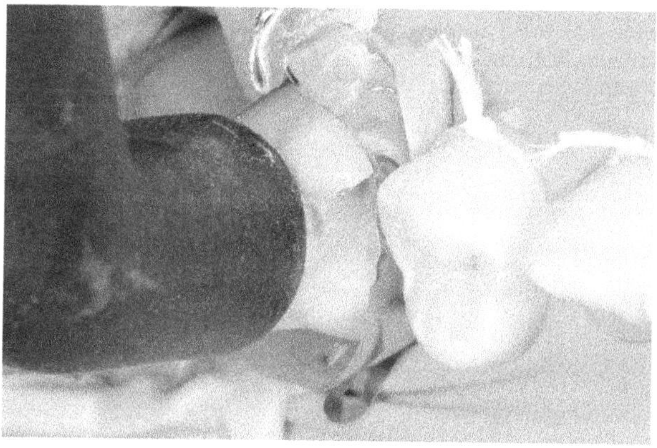

Fig. 8.25 Polymerization of the bonding during 20 s using a Demi Ultra unit

The cavity was restored using SonicFill 2 Unidose tips (shade A2) applied in one layer (Fig. 8.26). The composite was adapted using a ball spatula, sculpted, and polymerized for 40 s, using a powerful light curing device delivering at least 800 mW/cm^2 (Figs. 8.27 and 8.28). Following removal of the matrix, the proximal contour of the restoration was polished using the OptiDisc system to ensure an adequate and anatomical contact point between the two molars (Fig. 8.29). The same adhesive and restorative procedures were repeated for tooth 17, and Fig. 8.30 illustrates the two completed SonicFill 2 restorations prior to rubber dam removal.

Each restoration was finished and polished separately. After marking the occlusal excess and interferences with articulating paper, finishing was achieved using an egg-shaped fine diamond bur (Fig. 8.31). This was followed by a silicone point and a silicone filled brush (OccluBrush), resulting in a high lustre polish to the restorations (Figs. 8.32 and 8.33). Figure 8.34 shows a postoperative view of the final restorations after finishing and polishing. Figure 8.35 shows a digital radiograph of the two SonicFill 2 restorations, demonstrating perfect adaptation of the composite to the margins of the cavity with a higher degree of radiopacity of the composite material to that of enamel and dentine.

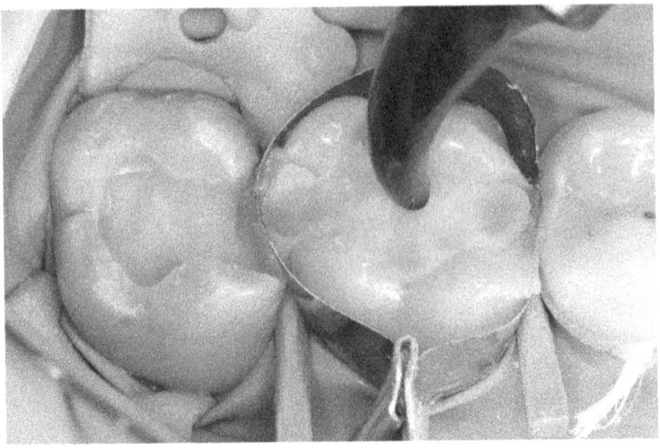

Fig. 8.26 Restoration of the cavity using one layer of Sonicfill 2 shade A2

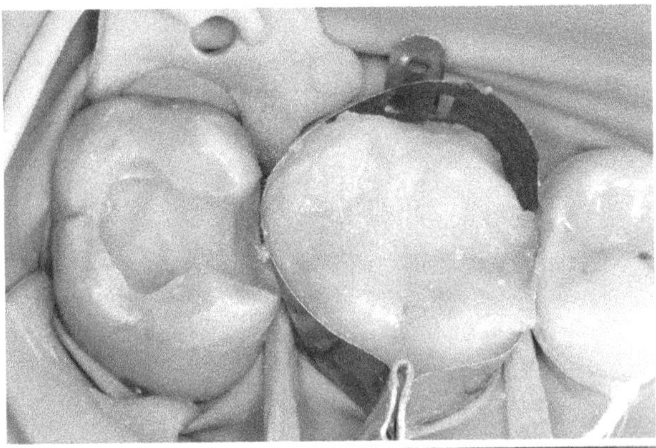

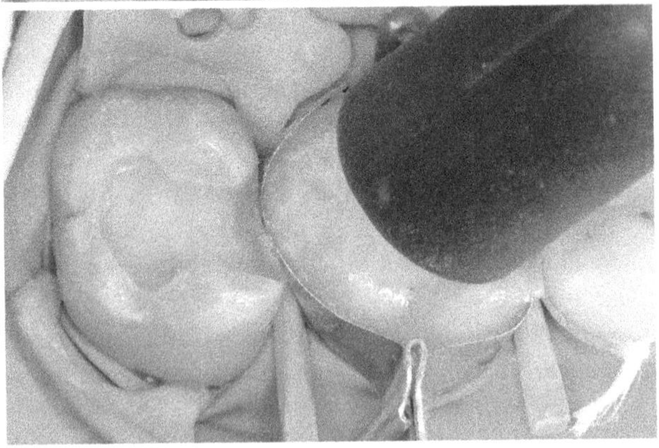

Figs. 8.27 and 8.28 Polymerization of the composite for 40 s

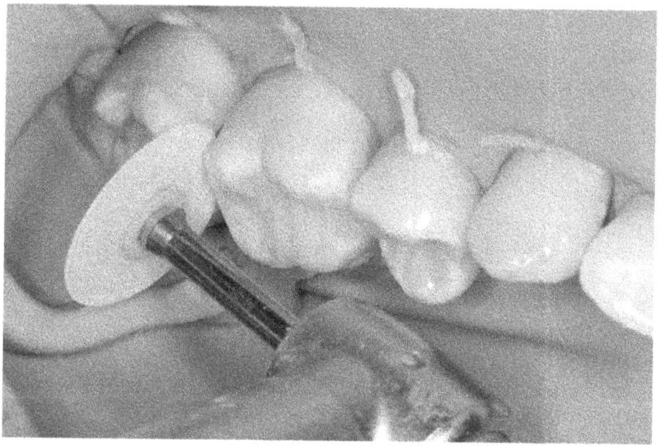

Fig. 8.29 Polishing of the proximal contour of the restoration using OptiDisc

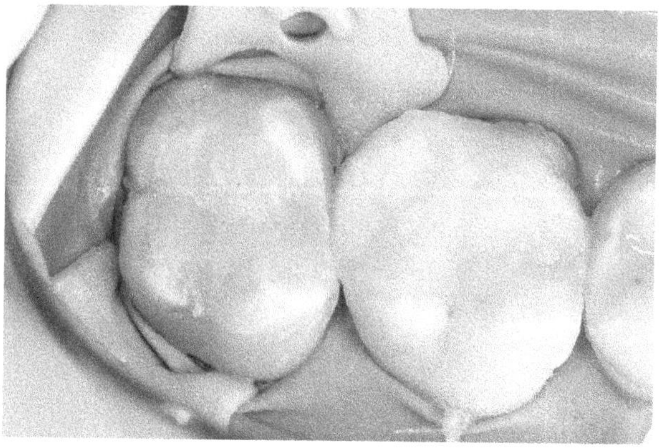

Fig. 8.30 The two completed SonicFill 2 restorations prior to rubber dam removal

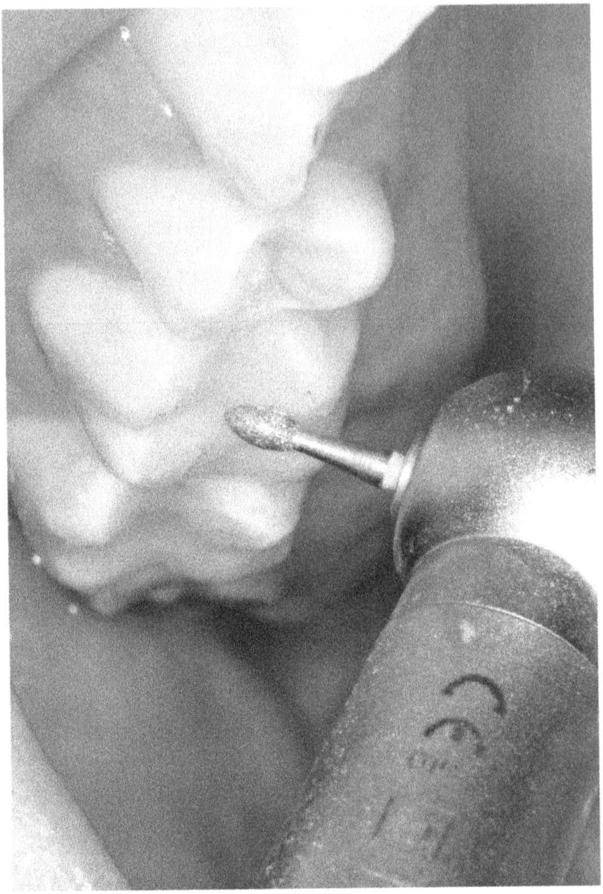

Fig. 8.31 Finishing of the composites with a fine egg shape diamond bur

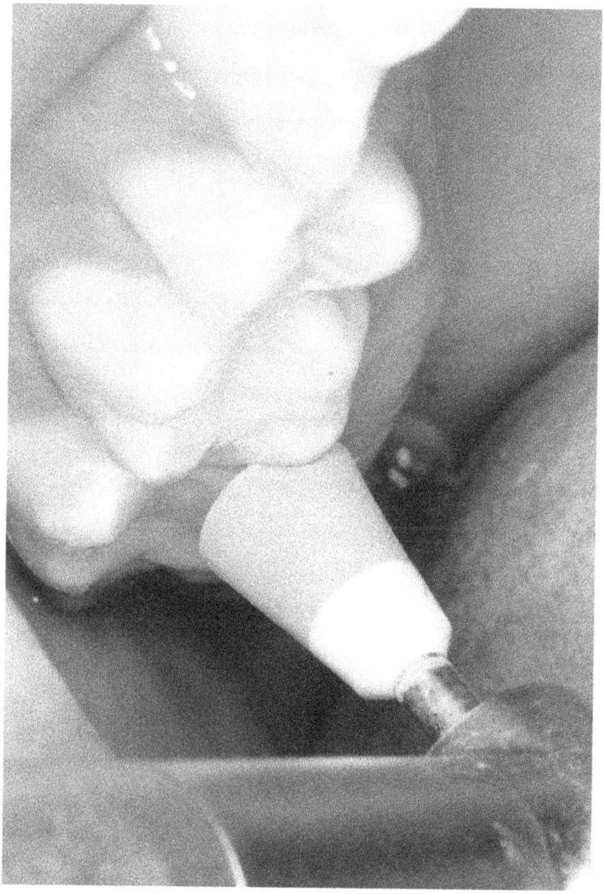

Fig. 8.32 Polishing of the restorations using a silicone point

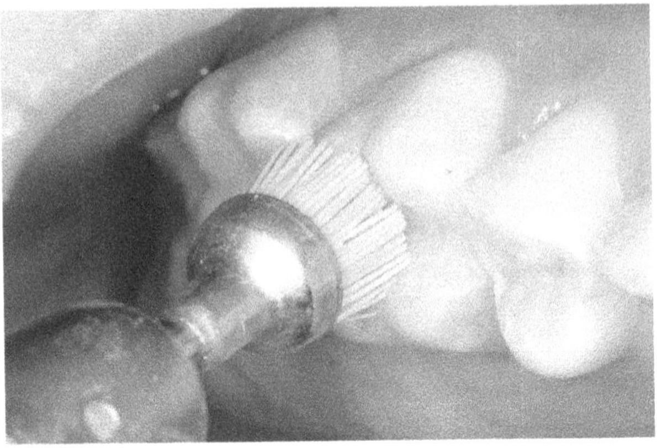

Fig. 8.33 Polishing of the restorations with Occlubrush

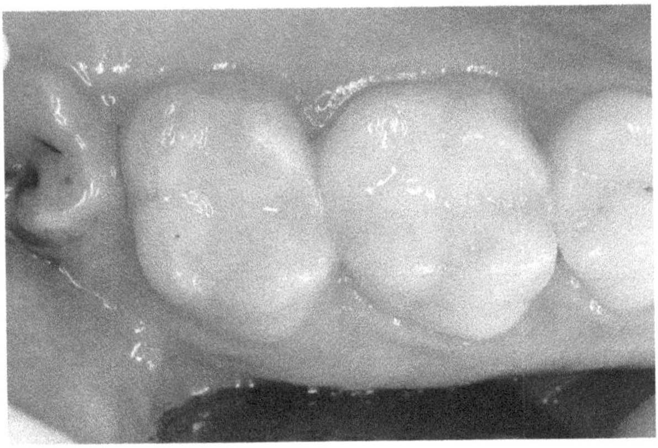

Fig. 8.34 Postoperative view of the finished Sonicfill 2 restorations

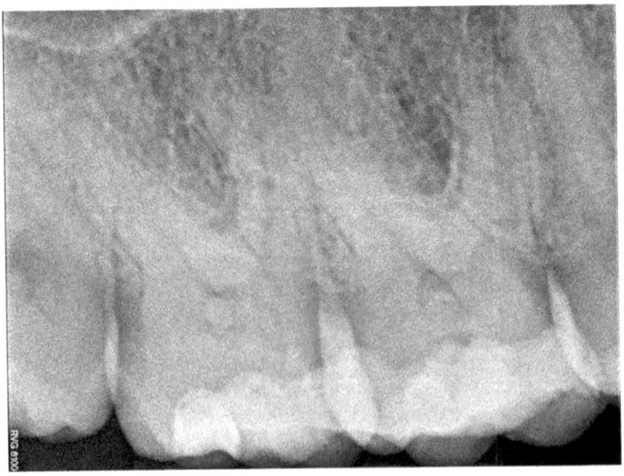

Fig. 8.35 Post-operative X-ray showing perfect adaptation of the restoration to the cavity

Case 8.4: Use of Highly Filled Bulk Fill Resin Composite, Filtek One Bulk Fill (3M-ESPE)
A 40-year-old patient presents complaining of sensitivity in the lower right arch, when drinking cold water or eating ice cream. The clinical exam revealed secondary caries under the existing amalgam restorations (Fig. 8.36).

Local anaesthesia was achieved, and caries was removed as described in the previous cases. After placement of the rubber dam, and a metallic matrix, etchant was applied (Fig. 8.37), followed by a fifth generation adhesive system (Scotchbond Universal) (Figs. 8.38 and 8.39).

A thin layer of opaque flowable composite (Essentia flow ML) was placed and polymerized on the floor of the cavity. This was applied to mask the dentin discoloration caused by the previous amalgam restoration (Figs. 8.40 and 8.41). The cavities were simultaneously restored using a highly filled bulk fill composite Filtek One Fill (3M-ESPE) (Figs. 8.42 and 8.43). The cavities were contoured, finished, and polished (Fig. 8.44). The pre-op and post-op radiographs demonstrate excellent adaptation of the new resin composite restorations and shows a radiopacity similar to enamel (Figs. 8.45 and 8.46).

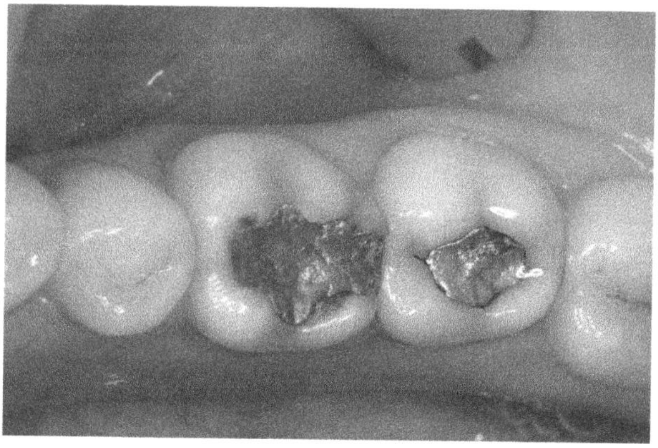

Fig. 8.36 Preoperative view of the restorations showing secondary caries under the existing amalgam restorations

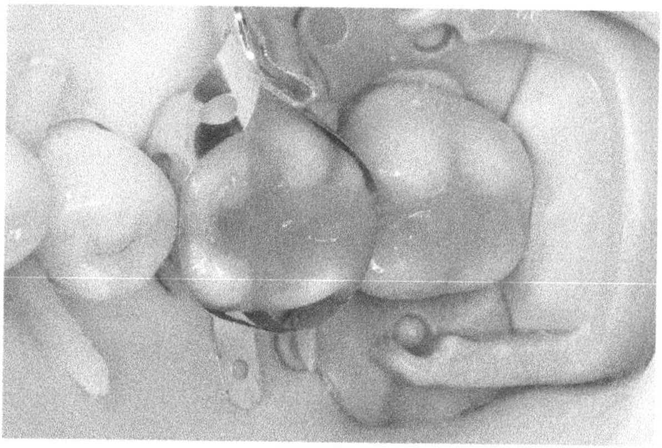

Fig. 8.37 Application of 37% phosphoric acid on enamel during 20 s after cavity isolation

Figs. 8.38 and 8.39 Application of the Scotchbond Universal adhesive on the cavity walls

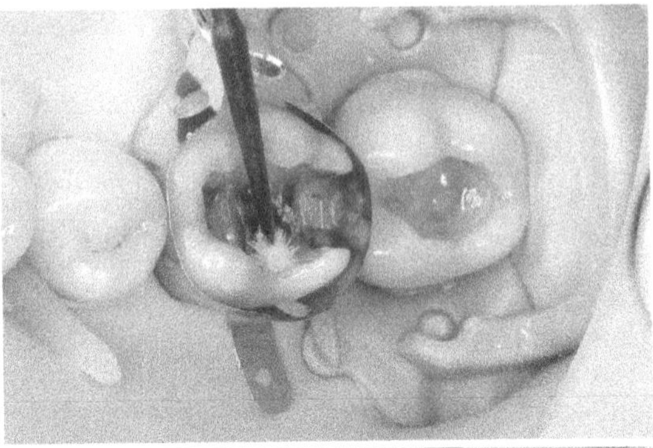

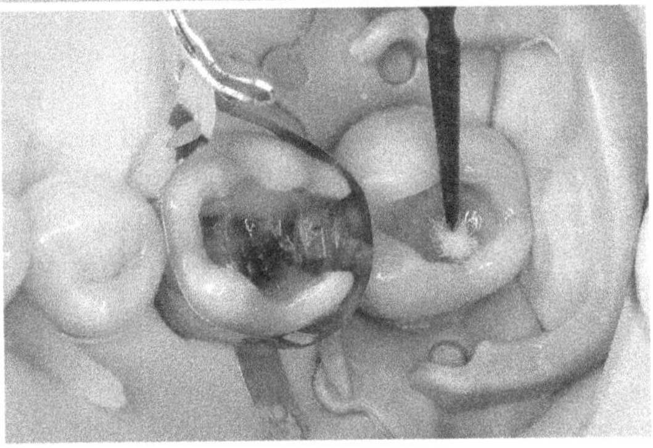

Figs. 8.40 and 8.41 Application of a thin layer of opaque flowable composite

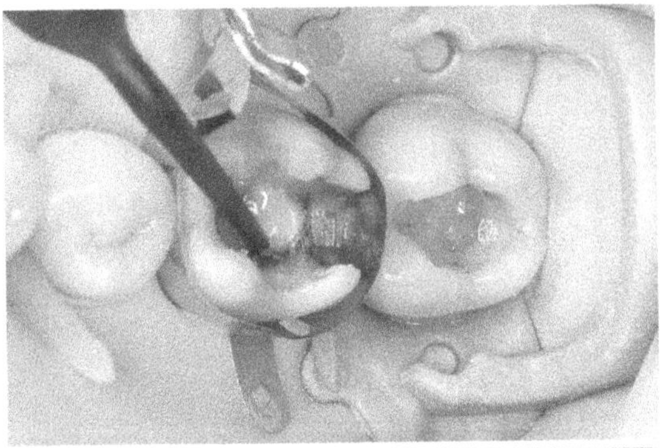

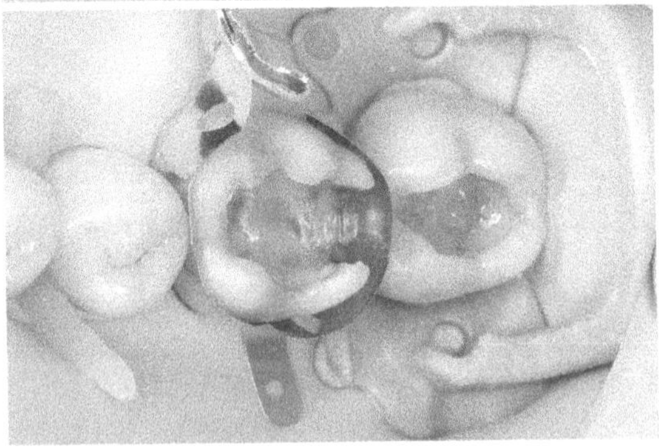

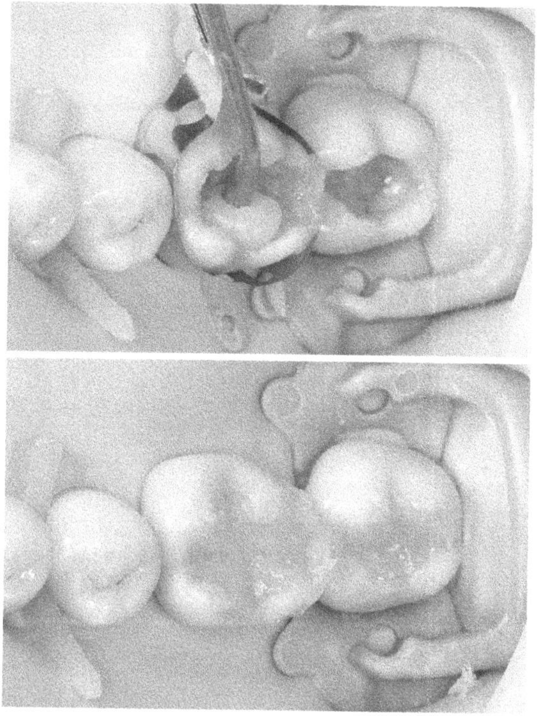

Figs. 8.42 and 8.43 Restoration of the cavity using a highly filled bulk fill composite Filtek One Fill (3M-ESPE)

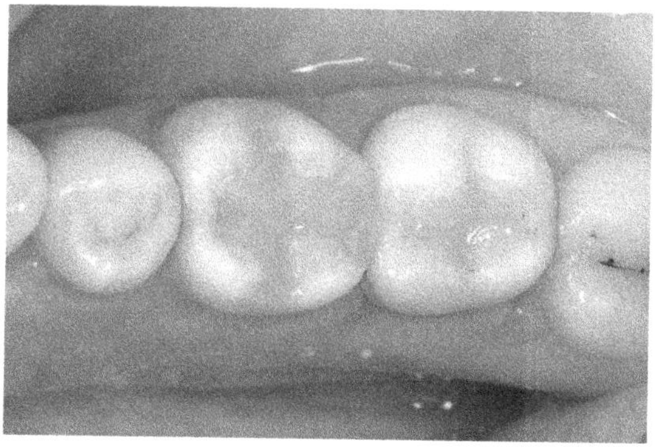

Fig. 8.44 Post-operative view of the cavities after finishing and polishing

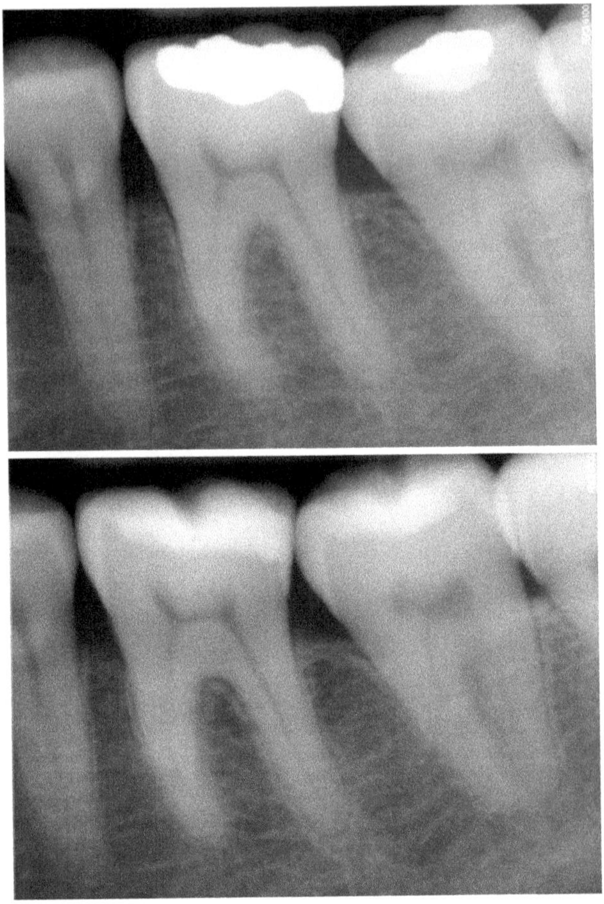

Figs. 8.45 and 8.46 Pre-op and post-op radiographs showing excellent adaptation of the bulk resin composite

Case 8.5: Use of the Centripetal Technique for Restoring a Class II Cavity
The centripetal technique is a method for creating a class II posterior restoration by replacing the lost interproximal tooth structure from the periphery towards the centre of the cavity. This achieves a better marginal adaptation to the gingival floor and a tight interproximal contact [16].

A patient presented with pain in lower first molar which had been previously restored with a resin composite material. A distal interproximal lesion was diagnosed (Fig. 8.47).

The caries was removed leaving as much enamel and dentine as possible (Fig. 8.48).

After placement of the rubber dam, and a metallic matrix, etchant was applied, followed by a fifth generation adhesive system (Scotchbond Universal) as previously discussed.

The missing proximal wall of the cavity is first restored with the restorative composite, converting the class II cavity into a class I cavity (Figs. 8.49–8.51).

This technique (centripetal) allows for the development of an excellent contact with the adjacent tooth and a good anatomically marginal ridge. It also gives better adaptation of the composite to the gingival floor and prevent microleakage [16].

The remaining of the class I cavity was filled, contoured, and finished (Figs. 8.52, 8.53, and 8.54).

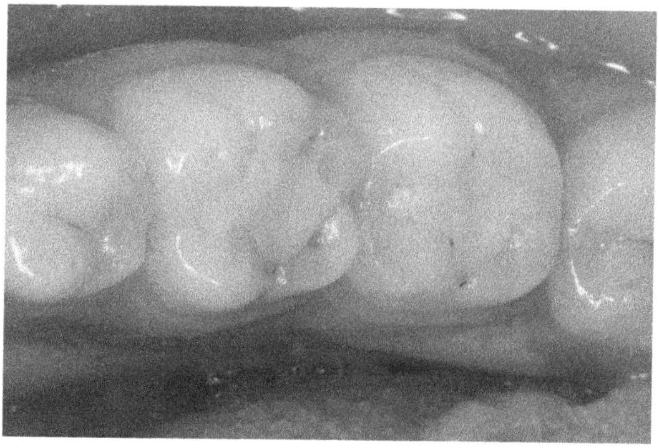

Fig. 8.47 Preoperative view of the first lower molar showing leakage around the margins

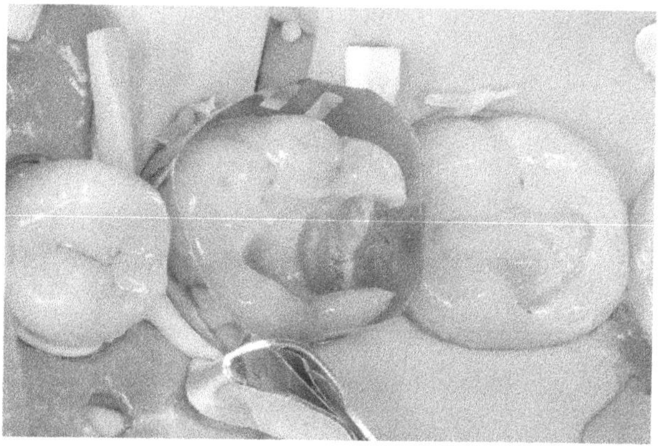

Fig. 8.48 Application of rubber dam after cavity preparation

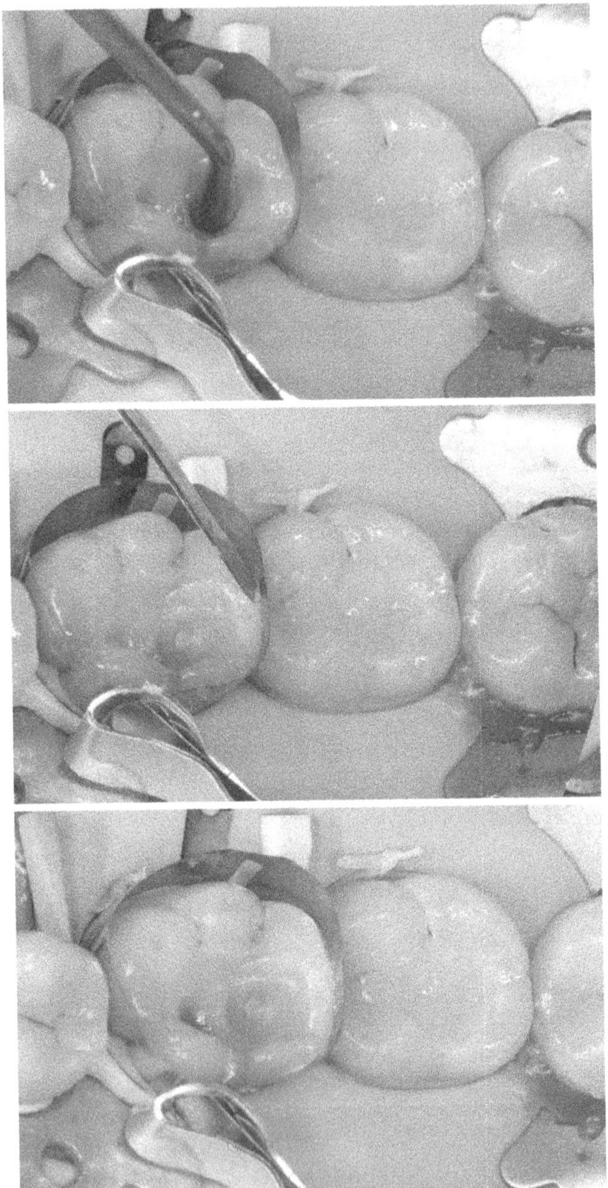

Figs. 8.49–8.51 Build-up of the proximal wall and conversion of the class II into class I

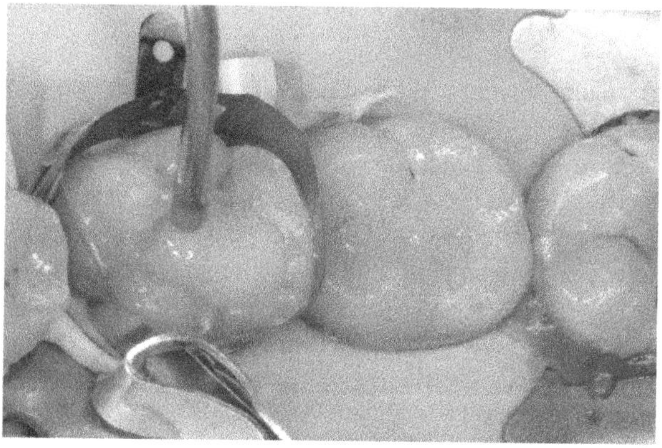

Fig. 8.52 Application of a layer of flowable bulk fill composite

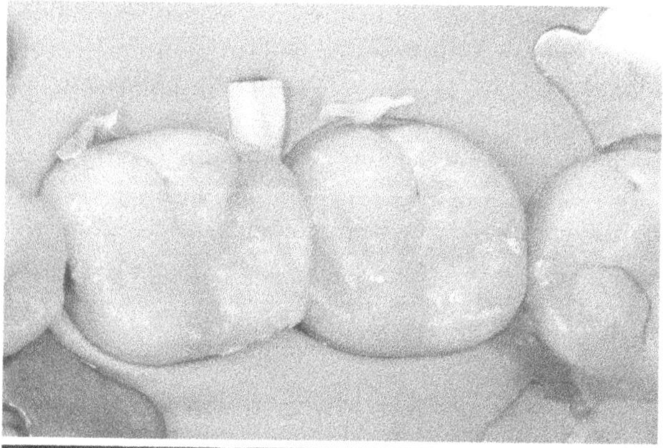

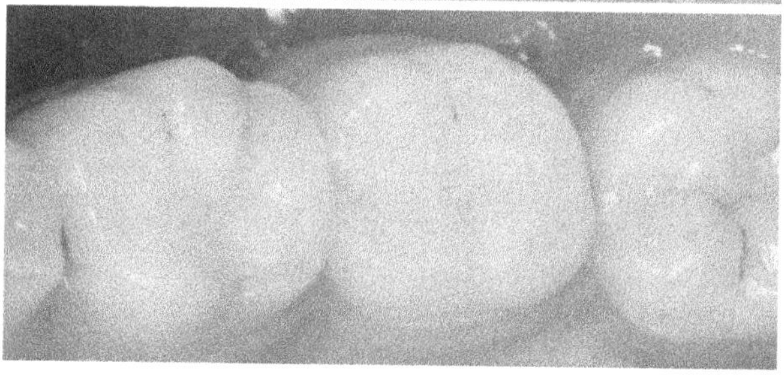

Figs. 8.53 and 8.54 Filling, contouring, and finishing of the class I cavities

8.5 Conclusion

Bulk fill posterior resin composites allows dentists a less stressful technique for restoring medium and large posterior cavities. Although they represent a heterogenous group of materials with different properties and clinical applications, bulk fill composites have shown similar clinical performance to conventional incremental composites in clinical trials. As already discussed in the previous chapters, restoration survival and annual failure rates are similar to conventional incremental composites.

The type and the quality of the light curing device used for BFC need to be optimal in terms of delivering enough energy for an optimal degree of conversion.

Flowable and fibre based bulk fill composites must be used according to the concept of closed sandwich technique where occlusal and proximal areas need to be protected by a conventional composite.

Sculptable bulk fill composites reduce restoration time, but the same has not been confirmed for flowable bulk fill and fibre-based materials, likely due to the required capping layer with a sculptable composite.

Challenges in clinical placement of bulk fill composites are the same as for composites, in general, and include moisture control, proper adhesive placement technique, material adaptation, and light curing. Diligence on the proper finishing and polishing of bulk fill posterior composites is essential.

References

1. Millar BJ. Principles and practice of esthetic dentistry-e-book: essentials of esthetic dentistry, vol. 1. Amsterdam: Elsevier Health Sciences; 2014.
2. Sabbagh J, Vreven J, Leloup G. Dynamic and static moduli of elasticity of resin-based materials. Dent Mater. 2002;18:64–71.
3. Ilie N, Hickel R. Investigations on a methacrylate-based flowable composite based on the SRD technology. Dent Mater. 2011;27:348–55.
4. Peumans M, Van Meerbeek B, Asscherickx K, Simon S, Abe Y, Lambrechts P, Vanherle G. Do condensable composites help to achieve better proximal contacts? Dent Mater. 2001;17(6):533–41.
5. Ziskind D, Adell I, Teperovich E, Peretz B. The effect of an intermediate layer of flowable resin composite on microleakage in packable composite restorations. Int J Paediatr Dent. 2005;15:349–54.
6. Efes BG, Dörter C, Gömec Y, Koray F. Two-year clinical evaluation of ormocer and nanofill composite with and without flowable liner. J Adhes Dent. 2006;8(2):119–25.
7. Ferracane JL, Lawson N. Probing the hierarchy of evidence to identify the best strategy for placing class II dental composite restorations using current materials. J Esthet Restor Dent. 2020;33:1–12.
8. Alqarni MA, Mathew VB, et al. Rubber dam isolation in clinical adhesive dentistry: the prevalence and assessment of associated radiolucencies. J Dent Res Rev. 2019;6:97–101.
9. Tardem C, Albuquerque EG, Lopes LDS, Marins SS, Calazans FS, Poubel LA, et al. Clinical time and postoperative sensitivity after use of bulk-fill (syringe and capsule) vs. incremental filling composites: a randomized clinical trial. Braz Oral Res. 2019;33:e089.

10. Bellinaso MD, Soares FZM, de Olivera Rocha R. Do bulk-fill resins decrease the restorative time in posterior teeth? A systematic review and meta-analysis of in vitro studies. J Investig Clin Dent. 2019;10(4):e12463.
11. Van Ende A, De Munck J, Lise DP, Van Meerbeek B. Bulk-fill composites: a review of the current literature. J Adhes Dent. 2017;19(2):95–109.
12. Sabbagh J, McConnell RJ, McConnell MC. Posterior composites: update on cavities and filling techniques. J Dent. 2017;57:86–90.
13. Leprince JG, Palin WM, Vanacker J, Sabbagh J, Devaux J, Leloup G. Physico-mechanical characteristics of commercially available bulk-fill composites. J Dent. 2014;42:993–1000.
14. Bucuta S, Ilie N. Light transmittance and micro-mechanical properties of bulk fill vs. conventional resin based composites. Clin Oral Investig. 2014;18:1991–2000.
15. Chesterman J, Jowett A, Gallacher A, Nixon P. Bulk-fill resin-based composite restorative materials: a review. Br Dent J. 2017;222:337–44.
16. Bichacho N. The centripetal build-up for composite resin posterior restorations. Pract Periodontics Aesthet Dent. 1994;6:17–23.
17. Tomaszewska IM, Kearns JO, Ilie N, Fleming GJ. Bulk fill restoratives: to cap or not to cap–that is the question? J Dent. 2015;43:309–16.
18. Quirynen M, Bollen CM. The influence of surface roughness and surface-free energy on supra- and subgingival plaque formation in man. J Clin Periodontol. 1995;22(1):1–14.
19. Shintani H, Satou J, Satou N, et al. Effects of various finishing methods on staining and accumulation of Streptococcus mutans HS-6 on resin composites. Dent Mater. 1985;1(6): 225–7.
20. Reis AF, Giannini M, Lovadino JR, Ambrosano GM. Effects of various finishing systems on the surface roughness and staining susceptibility of packable resin composites. Dent Mater. 2003;19(1):12–8.
21. Bollen CM, Lambrechts P, Quirynen M. Comparison of surface roughness of oral hard materials to the threshold surface roughness for bacterial plaque retention: a review of the literature. Dent Mater. 1997;13(4):258–69.
22. Cazzaniga G, Ottobelli M, Ionescu AC, Paolone G, Gherlone E, Ferracane JL, Brambilla E. In vitro biofilm formation on resin-based composites after different finishing and polishing procedures. J Dent. 2017;67:43–52.
23. Strassler HE, Baum G. Current concepts in polishing resin composites. Pract Periodontics Aesthet Dent. 1993;5(3 Supplement 1):12–7.
24. Yap AU, Lye KW, Sau CW. Surface characteristics of tooth-colored restoratives polished utilizing different polishing systems. Oper Dent. 1997;22(6):260–5.
25. Antonson SA, Yazici AR, Kilinc E, et al. Comparison of different finishing/ polishing systems on surface roughness and gloss of resin composites. J Dent. 2011;39(Supplement 1):e9–e17.
26. Attar N. The effect of finishing and polishing procedures on the surface roughness of resin composite materials. J Contemp Dent Pract. 2007;8(1):27–35.
27. Güler AU, Güler E, Yücel AC, Ertaş E. Effects of polishing procedures on color stability of resin composites. J Appl Oral Sci. 2009;17(2):108–12.
28. Da Costa J, Ferracane J, Paravina RD, et al. The effect of different polishing systems on surface roughness and gloss of various resin composites. J Esthet Restor Dent. 2007;19(4):214–26.
29. O'Neill C, Kreplak L, Rueggeberg FA, et al. Effect of tooth brushing on gloss retention and surface roughness of five bulk-fill resin composites. J Esthet Restor Dent. 2018;30(1):59–69.
30. Rigo LC, Bordin D, Fardin VP, et al. Influence of polishing system on the surface roughness of flowable and regular-viscosity bulk fill composites. Int J Periodontics Restorative Dent. 2018;38(4):e79–86.
31. Lawson NC, Burgess JO. Gloss and stain resistance of ceramic-polymer CAD/CAM restorative blocks. J Esthet Restor Dent. 2016;28(Suppl 1):S40–5.
32. Vichi A, Louca C, Corciolani G, Ferrari M. Color related to ceramic and zirconia restorations: a review. Dent Mater. 2011;27(1):97–108.

33. Vichi A, Fabian Fonzar R, et al. Effect of finishing and polishing on roughness and gloss of lithium disilicate and lithium silicate zirconia reinforced glass ceramic for CAD/CAM systems. Oper Dent. 2018;43(1):90–100.
34. Lee YK, Lu H, Oguri M, Powers JM. Changes in gloss after simulated generalized wear of resin composites. J Prosthet Dent. 2005;94(4):370–6.
35. Lee YK, Lim BS, Rhee SH, et al. Color and translucency of A2 shade resin composites after curing, polishing and thermocycling. Oper Dent. 2005;30(4):436–42.
36. Paolone G, Moratti E, Goracci C, Gherlone E, Vichi A. Effect of finishing systems on surface roughness and gloss of full-body bulk-fill resin composites. Materials (Basel). 2020;13(24):5657.
37. Willems G, Lambrechts P, Braem M, et al. The surface roughness of enamel-to-enamel contact areas compared with the intrinsic roughness of dental resin composites. J Dent Res. 1991;70(9):1299–305.
38. Mörmann WH, Stawarczyk B, Ender A, et al. Wear characteristics of current aesthetic dental restorative CAD/CAM materials: two-body wear, gloss retention, roughness and martens hardness. J Mech Behav Biomed Mater. 2013;20:113–25.
39. Barucci-Pfister N, Göhring TN. Subjective and objective perceptions of specular gloss and surface roughness of esthetic resin composites before and after artificial aging. Am J Dent. 2009;22(2):102–10.
40. Silikas N, Kavvadia K, Eliades G, Watts D. Surface characterization of modern resin composites: a multitechnique approach. Am J Dent. 2005;18(2):95–100.
41. Cook MP, Thomas K. Evaluation of glossmeters for measurement of moulded plastics. Polym Test. 1990;9:233–44.
42. Garoushi S, Lassila LV, Tezvergil A, Vallittu PK. Load bearing capacity of fiber-reinforced and particulate filler resin composite combination. J Dent. 2006;34:179–84.
43. Garoushi S, Lassila LVJ, Tezvergil A, Vallittu PK. Static and fatigue compression test for particulate filler resin composite with fiber-reinforced composite substructure. Dent Mater. 2007;23:17.

9 Clinical Challenges and Longevity of Bulk-Fill Materials

Vesna Miletic

9.1 Introduction

Clinical application of composites in increments thicker than 2 mm began in 2003, when QuiXfil (Dentsply) appeared on the market and in dental practice. The manufacturer's recommended increment thickness for this material was 4 mm. The true clinical era of "bulk-fill" composite materials began when Smart Dentin Replacement (SDR, Dentsply) was launched in 2009.

Scientific evidence has shown comparable polymerization shrinkage and stress [1], depth of cure [2, 3], physico-mechanical properties [4–6] and marginal adaptation [6–8] of bulk-fill and universal composites. In vitro data indicate that these materials may be used as recommended for dentin replacement in posterior teeth in increments up to 4–5 mm (flowable bulk-fill) or as full restorations (sculptable bulk-fill) in posterior cavities without cusp replacement [9].

Within the last decade, all major manufacturers have at least one bulk-fill composite in their portfolio, and many have several types of bulk-fills (flowable and sculptable) as well as second "generation" of the original material. Bulk-fill composites were expected to reduce clinical working time as fewer increments are needed to restore posterior cavities compared to universal composites recommended for 2 mm increments. Indeed, a recent meta-analysis by Bellinaso et al. [10] confirmed that sculptable ("full-body") bulk-fill composites shorten restorative time in posterior teeth compared to conventional composites. The same, however, was not found for flowable bulk-fill composites. The true value of these findings should be verified in further research, as only three studies with moderate to substantial heterogeneity were included in the above meta-analysis [10]. Nevertheless, scientific

V. Miletic (✉)
Faculty of Medicine and Health, Sydney Dental School, The University of Sydney, Sydney, NSW, Australia
e-mail: vesna.miletic@sydney.edu.au

J. Sabbagh, R. McConnell (eds.), *Bulk Fill Resin Composites in Dentistry*,
https://doi.org/10.1007/978-3-031-16388-3_9

and clinical interest in these materials and continuous improvements reflect the potential of bulk-fill composites to alter clinical practice related to posterior restorations.

9.2 Criteria for Clinical Evaluation of Restorative Materials

Clinical performance of bulk-fill composites, as well as restorative materials in general is evaluated using either of the following sets of criteria: (1) modified USPHS[1] and (2) FDI.[2]

Modified USPHS are based on evaluation criteria published by Cvar and Ryge [11] in 1971, which initially used five categories of esthetic and functional performance: color match, cavosurface marginal discoloration, anatomic form, marginal adaptation and caries. The ratings, as originally presented by Cvar and Ryge, include a series of bipolar decisions as "Yes"/"No" answers to questions specific for a certain criterion until a code is reached. The Cvar and Ryge criteria were expanded in 1980 by a panel of researchers to include more categories, such as post-operative sensitivity, occlusion, fracture and retention. These criteria are known as "modified USPHS" criteria [12]. The ratings or scores in modified USPHS criteria indicate progressively less acceptable performance from "Alpha"—clinically ideal situation, "Bravo"—minor deviations from norm but clinically acceptable, "Charlie"—unacceptable deviation from norm requiring re-intervention to prevent future damage to "Delta"—unacceptable deviation from norm requiring immediate replacement. Some studies use numerical scores (e.g., 0–4) to indicate ratings, with 0 corresponding to an ideal clinical situation to 4 indicating clinically unacceptable rating [13, 14]. Definitions of each score for each evaluation criterion vary in different clinical trials [15–20]. Confusion may be further created when referencing the original Cvar and Ryge criteria and claiming that modified USPHS criteria were used as the latter is a broader set. This is especially so when a non-original criterion (e.g. surface roughness/texture) is used without proper score definition [21, 22]. Therefore, it is recommended to state the criteria and define the scores/ratings when reporting clinical trials because of the lack of uniformity in modified USPSHS criteria [12]. A summary of variations in score definitions in clinical trials on bulk-fill composites using modified USPHS criteria is presented in a recent meta-analysis by Veloso et al. [23].

A more comprehensive and discriminatory evaluation system, known as FDI clinical criteria, was introduced in 2007 [24] and updated in 2010 [25]. This system is based on three sets of criteria: esthetic, functional and biological. Each set contains a subset of criteria (16 in total) with 5 scores: (1) clinically excellent/very good—ideal clinical situation; (2) clinically good—minor deviation from the norm; (3) clinically sufficient/satisfactory—minor shortcomings, no unacceptable effects but not adjustable without damage to the tooth; (4)—clinically unsatisfactory but repairable and (5) clinically poor—replacement necessary. Scores 4 and 5 are

[1] United States Public Health Service.

[2] World Dental Federation (Fédération Dentaire Internationale).

considered relative and absolute failures, respectively [25]. The former score indicates repaired existing restorations while the latter indicates replacement as the existing restoration is beyond repairable. Hickel et al. [25] recommend that selected FDI criteria may be used in clinical trials instead of the entire set of 16 criteria, depending on the trial objective. Furthermore, they recommend that five scores may be reduced to 4 or even 2, depending on the purpose of the study and the tested material or procedure. This should be carefully considered as reduced scores may result in lower discriminatory power of evaluation, similar to modified USPHS criteria. A recent randomized clinical trial (RCT) comparing two bulk-fill composites to a conventional control composite found significant differences between modified USPHS and FDI scores in that FDI scores were mostly "success" while USPHS were mostly "acceptable" [16].

Both "modified USPHS" and "FDI criteria" rely on subjective examiners' judgment. To reduce the risk of bias and ensure consistency, clinical evaluation is conducted independently by at least two trained or calibrated examiners. Consistency in judgment is of critical importance for valid evaluation. Inter-examiner agreement is agreement between different examiners and intra-examiner agreement relates to agreement of one examiner's judgment on different occasions. An inter-examiner and intra-examiner agreement of at least 85% is considered acceptable [11]. For training purposes, photographs, radiographs and models are useful in anchoring definitions related to specific characteristics. In the internet era, online databases may serve as excellent training and calibration resources. One example was e-calib.info, an online database developed in 2008, which contained about 300 high quality clinical photographs. This database was used to train and calibrate examiners in 8 of 16 FDI criteria. Unfortunately, e-calib database is no longer accessible. Another potential solution is development of digital and laser-based evaluation techniques to improve standardization and avoid bias. Expansion of intraoral scanners and software solutions allow high quality reproduction of teeth and restorations and could be used for, at least, some aspects of clinical evaluation, e.g. luster, staining, color match and translucency, anatomic form, marginal adaptation, contour and wear.

9.3 Clinical Performance of Bulk-Fill Composites

One of the first randomized control trials (RCTs) compared performance of an early sculptable bulk-fill material (QuiXfil, Dentsply) to a hybrid composite (Tetric Ceram, Ivoclar) with their respective adhesive systems. Comparable results between the two composites were reported at 3 years with significantly worse results for marginal discoloration and integrity of QuiXfil and marginal discoloration of Tetric Ceram [26]. At 10 years, 26 QuiXfil and 30 Tetric Ceram restorations were evaluated out of the initial 46 and 50, respectively. The main reasons for failure were secondary caries and marginal discoloration, followed by tooth fracture, restoration fracture, post-operative sensitivity and deterioration of the marginal integrity [27]. Overall, the control material Tetric Ceram performed slightly better than the bulk-fill QuiXfil in terms of the overall annual failure rate (1.6% vs. 2.5%, respectively) and success rate (86.7% vs. 76.9%, respectively) but the difference did not reach statistical significance [27]. Statistical significance was related to cavity/restoration size, i.e. large restorations failed significantly more often than small restorations [27]. To date, this is the only RCT comparing bulk-fill and conventional composites with 10 years follow-up.

9.3.1 Systematic Reviews and Meta-Analyses

Clinical trials on bulk-fill composites increased as of 2014, with annual numbers of published clinical trials rising steadily over the past couple of years. Beside randomized clinical trials (RCTs), several systematic reviews and meta-analyses were published in the last 3 years, comparing clinical effectiveness of bulk-fill to conventional methacrylate-based composites [1, 10, 23, 28, 29].

Arbildo-Vega et al. [28] included 16 unique RCTs with follow-up periods from 6 months to 10 years in which sculptable bulk-fill, flowable and sculptable two-step restorations were compared to conventional incremental composites. Clinical effectiveness of bulk-fills was found to be similar to conventional composites, regardless of the type of restoration (class I, II, or non-carious cervical lesions), the type of tooth restored (primary or permanent teeth), or the restoration technique used (incremental, bulk, or two-step bulk) [28]. In terms of fractures, marginal staining and adaptation, secondary caries, color stability and translucency, surface texture and anatomical form, no significant differences were found between conventional and bulk-fill composites. In terms of post-operative sensitivity, the meta-analysis found no difference between conventional and two-step bulk restorations. However, reduced or no post-operative sensitivity was associated with conventional materials in non-carious cervical lesions as well as incremental technique in permanent dentition.

Cidreira Boaro et al. [1] included 11 RCTs spanning from 12 months to 10 years. No significant difference in clinical performance of bulk-fill and conventional composites was reported. In addition to RCTs, this meta-analysis included 137 other in vitro studies comparing an array of material properties. Polymerization stress and cusp deflection were found to be significantly lower in bulk-fill composites. No differences were found between bulk-fill and conventional composites regarding flexural and fracture strength. As for volumetric shrinkage, microhardness and degree of conversion, the results varied depended on material viscosity and specimen thickness. Differences in the above-mentioned properties detected in vitro did not result in differences in clinical performance of bulk-fill and conventional composites. It should be highlighted that only 1 RCT was evaluated for each of the follow-up periods of 5, 6 and 10 years with the majority of RCTs reporting for 1-year follow-up [1].

Veloso et al. [23] included 10 RCTs with follow-up periods between 1 and 6 years. No significant difference in clinical performance was found between bulk-fill and conventional composites, irrespective of the viscosity of the bulk-fill material (sculptable or flowable requiring a capping layer). Failure rates were 5.57% (29 of 520) in bulk-fill and 3.32% (14 of 421) in conventional composites. The causes of restoration failure were reported to be secondary caries (23%), tooth and resin fractures (19% each), post-operative sensitivity (9%), anatomical shape and marginal adaptation (7%), marginal discoloration (9%), caries associated with tooth fracture (5%) and retention (2%).

Kruly et al. [29] conducted a meta-analysis on various types of composites, comparing non-conventional (ormocer, silorane and bulk-fill) to conventional methacrylate-based composites. Bulk-fills were investigated in three studies of the 21 studies included in the review with 1–3 years follow-up periods. All non-conventional composites were grouped when evaluating post-operative sensitivity, secondary caries, retention, marginal adaptation and discoloration, so no conclusion was made specifically for bulk-fill materials as a separate group. Restorations conducted with low polymerization shrinkage composites, such as silorane, ormocer and bulk-fill type showed clinical performance similar to restorations with conventional methacrylate-based composites [29].

According to Hickel et al. [24] restoration failures are classified as early (0–6 months), medium time frame (6–24 months) and long-term (beyond 18 or 24 months). The majority of RCTs evaluated in meta-analyses reported findings at 12 months follow-up with progressively fewer studies reporting after longer follow-up periods [1, 23, 28], hence detecting to a greater extent only short- to medium-time failures.

All meta-analyses expressed the need for long-term properly designed RCTs following the CONSORT 2010 statement [30]. This 25-item checklist and a flow diagram ensure transparency and completeness in reporting RCTs. Though CONSORT only focuses on reporting with no specific recommendations on study design, conduct and data analysis, it indirectly affects design and implementation by including specific items such as participant eligibility criteria, sample size calculation, allocation sequencing, primary and secondary outcomes with information on how and when they were assessed.

Sample size calculation, randomization, allocation concealment and blinding have been identified in meta-analyses on bulk-fill composites as characteristics that increase the risk of bias. Operator blinding is not possible due to different clinical protocols for bulk-fill and conventional composites, but patient and outcome assessment blinding should be implemented to avoid bias.

In reporting interventions in restorative dentistry additional factors need to be considered in study design and reporting. These were summarized in Hickel et al. [24]:

1. Patient's oral status (including pre-existent damage to the tooth), attitudes, habits.
2. Participant selection reflective of population at large.
3. Limit the split-mouth design to one test and one control restoration.
4. Detailed description of the restorative procedure (cavity type and size, bevelling, lining, adhesives, composites, light-curing, finishing and polishing procedures).
5. Evaluation to be performed by calibrated evaluators independent of personal or situational bias.

6. Confounding factors to be controlled by inclusion/exclusion criteria (for patients, teeth, operators), randomization, matching the confounding variable and/or including it in statistical analysis.

9.3.2 Recent Randomized Clinical Trials and Other Clinical Trials

Several randomized clinical trials (RCTs) were published around or after the latest meta-analysis [28] and, hence, were not included in this review. The same search strategy as the one used in the most recent meta-analysis by Arbildo-Vega et al. [28] was applied to identify more recent RCTs, i.e. those published around the same time or after the latest systematic review and meta-analysis [28]. The same databases (PubMED, CENTRAL, Web of Science, Scopus and EMBASE) were searched using the same keywords: ("dental caries" or "dental restoration, permanent") AND ("bulk fill" or "bulk fill" or "bulk-fill" or "bulk") AND ("composite resins" or "composite resin" or "resin composite" or "resin composites" or "resin restoration" or "composite restoration" or "composite restorations").

A total of 1230 studies were retrieved from database search up until July 2021. The search was then modified to include the keyword "clinical" in all fields to narrow the search and avoid unnecessary screening of non-clinical trials. It is self-evident that any type of clinical trial, especially RCTs, must contain this word in either title, abstract or the keywords. This resulted in 642 results. After screening for duplicates and removal of studies that were not clinical trials, 51 studies were assessed for eligibility based on inclusion and exclusion criteria.

Inclusion criteria were: (1) Studies carried out on permanent vital teeth in human participants; (2) RCTs comparing bulk-fill and conventional composites and (3) Prospective clinical studies evaluating bulk-fill composites. These inclusion criteria allowed inclusion of not only RCTs but also other prospective clinical trials as the aim was to provide a comprehensive narrative review and not conduct another meta-analysis. This approach allowed wider inclusion of studies, some of which would be excluded in a meta-analytical approach, despite presenting relevant clinical information.

Exclusion criteria were: (1) Studies on primary teeth; (2) Studies involving pulpotomy or root canal treatment; (3) Retrospective studies; (4) Insights, letters to editor, article review; (5) The same studies at different times; (6) Studies already included in meta-analyses; (7) Studies in a language other than English and where full text was unavailable.

Finally, 16 studies were found eligible and included in further analysis. Literature review and selection process are shown in Fig. 9.1.

Table 9.1 summarizes the main characteristics of these reviewed clinical trials (See Appendix 1). Eight studies are RCTs comparing bulk-fill and conventional incremental composites in a split-mouth design [16, 17, 21, 31–35], five are RCTs evaluating only bulk-fill composites with a different test group [36–40], one is an RCT that compared bulk-fill and incremental composites but in parallel-group

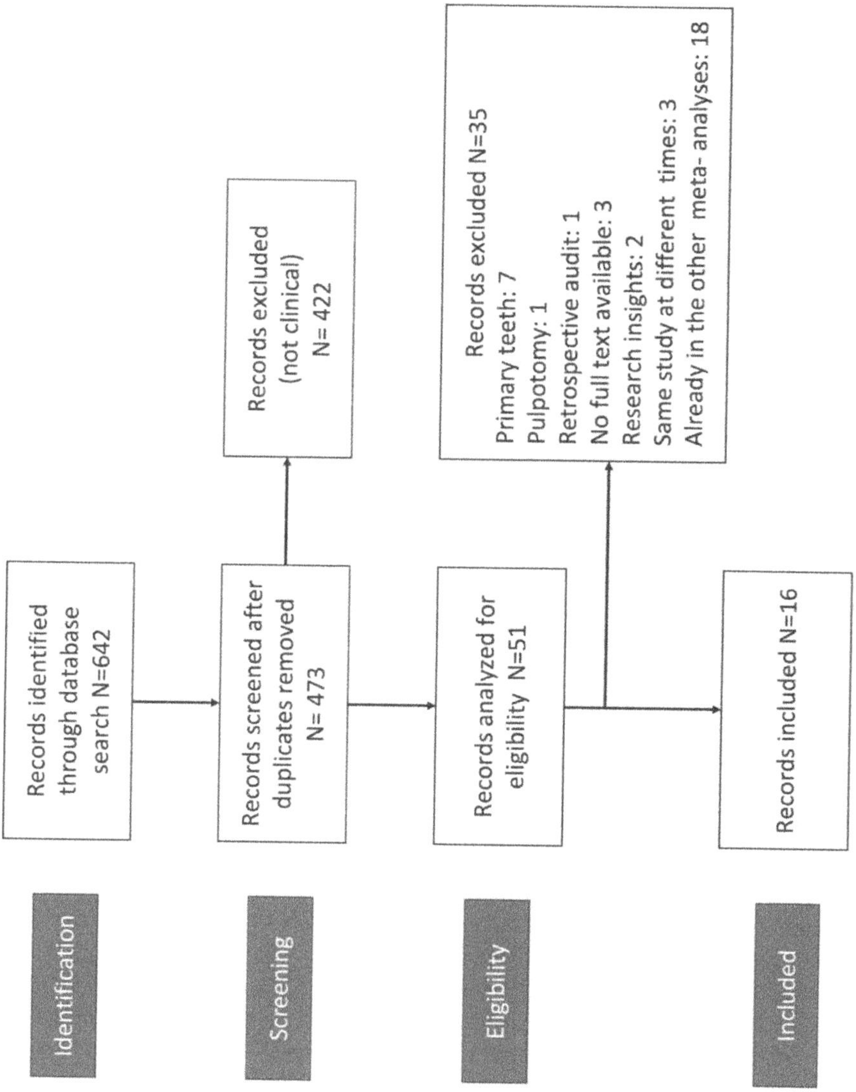

Fig. 9.1 PRISMA search flow diagram

design and only evaluating post-operative sensitivity [25] and two studies were prospective clinical trials with only a bulk-fill test group without a control group [15, 20].

The overall success or survival rate of bulk-fill composites ranged from 100% [18, 32, 33, 36, 39] and 97.1% [17] to 88.1% [37] at 12 months, 100% [40] to 99.1% at 2 years [15], 100% [38] to 94.44% with an annual failure rate of 1.26% at 3 years follow-up [16], 94.28% [21] to 93.9% with annual failure rates of 0.95% [21] to 1% [14] at 6 years. At 10 years, overall success rates of a bulk-fill and conventional composite were 76.9% and 86.7%, respectively, with an overall annual failure rate of 2.5% for the bulk-fill and 1.6% for the conventional composite [27]. Reasons for failure were recurrent caries, unacceptable marginal adaptation [16], pulpal or periapical inflammation [15, 17], crown replacement (no reason provided) [21] and "lost restoration" (no reason provided) [37].

Similar clinical performance in terms of esthetic, functional and biological FDI criteria was reported for ormocer bulk-fill composite (Admira Fusion x-tra, Voco) compared to the conventional, incremental ormocer (Admira Fusion, Voco) at 2 years [35]. Placement of sculptable bulk-fill composites required less chair time than incremental placement [34, 35].

In most randomized clinical trials (RCTs), the majority of criteria were comparable irrespective of the evaluation method (modified USPSH or FDI). There were little differences between bulk-fill and conventional control composites, somewhat lower incidence, intensity and duration of post-operative sensitivity [31], lower pain and marginal discoloration in the bulk-fill group at 12 months [33], lower marginal discoloration in the bulk-fill at 6 years though both bulk-fill and conventional composite exhibited significant deterioration in marginal discoloration compared to baseline [21], surface luster in one of the two tested bulk-fills compared to a conventional control at 3 years [41], marginal integrity but worse in color match than conventional composite onlays [17]. The overall risk for post-operative sensitivity was found to be 4% and significantly greater within the first 48 h post-restoration [34]. This overall risk for post-operative sensitivity was found to be independent of material (bulk vs. conventional), adhesive strategy (total-etch vs. self-etch) or delivery method (capsule vs. syringe) but was found to be significantly higher in cavities deeper than 4 mm [34]. Similarly, post-operative pain was mostly recorded within the first 48 h post-restoration in another study that compared different placement and bonding techniques and only used one bulk-fill composite [42]. This is the same study as [38] but only reporting on post-operative sensitivity. However, unlike in [34], Costa et al. [42] reported an overall risk of post-operative sensitivity of 20.3%. Cavities with 3–4 surfaces were significantly more at risk of post-operative pain that 1–2 surface cavities. Adhesive strategy or composite placement technique had no effect on incidence or intensity of post-operative pain. Differences between these studies in the risk of post-operative sensitivity warrant further research, especially taking into account factor operator.

Several RCTs compared clinical performance of bulk-fill composites in both the test and control group, but with different placement techniques (bulk vs. incremental) [38, 39], bonding techniques (wet vs. dry bonding of a 2-step total-etch [36] or total-etch vs. self-etch adhesive [38]), with or without a lining material [40] or cured with a high-intensity vs. low-intensity light-curing units [37]. In general, comparable performance was reported in short- and medium-time frame of 12–36 months. Significantly greater percentage of marginal discontinuity involving occlusal margins at 12 months was reported for "high-intensity" than "low-intensity" light-curing group [37]. In another study, marginal staining and adaptation at 36 months were found to be significantly worse when a bulk-fill composite was used with a self-etch than total-etch adhesive [38].

Distinct, statistically significant differences were found in an RCT comparing a sculptable bulk-fill composite (Filtek One Bulk Fill, 3M) and a self-adhesive bulk-fill composite (SABF, 3M) with more unfavorable scores for the latter in terms of surface luster, marginal staining and color match already at 12 months [32]. The self-adhesive bulk-fill composite is intended for use without an adhesive system due to the presence of a phosphoric acid functionalized methacrylate. Manufacturer's instructions recommend mixing for 15 s, placing in one bulk increment in unconditioned cavities and light-curing albeit the material is dual-curing and hence allows only limited sculpting time during auto-polymerization. These initial results indicate inferior esthetic performance of the self-adhesive bulk-fill to other bulk-fill and conventional composites. Its unfavorable marginal staining as early as 12 months post-restoration indicates inability of the phosphoric acid functionalized methacrylate in this self-adhesive composite to substitute an adhesive system.

Recent RCTs present a positive trend in that the split-mouth design is a predominant form of clinical trials evaluating bulk-fill composites. When appropriately designed and conducted, RCTs represent a gold-standard in evaluating healthcare interventions [30]. The split-mouth approach eliminates a number of factors potentially affecting the restorations, i.e. caries risk, oral hygiene, dietary habits, masticatory characteristics, bruxism, etc. In the majority of studies, the split-mouth design involved placement of 1 test and 1 control restoration [17, 21, 32, 33, 35–37, 39, 40, 43], albeit in some cases more than 1 pair of restorations was placed per patient [16, 31, 34, 38].

Progress can be seen in recent clinical trials on bulk-fill composites with regard to study design characteristics identified as limitations in previous meta-analyses. Sample size calculation, randomization, allocation concealment and blinding were all included in study design and reported in the majority of studies [16, 17, 21, 31, 34–36, 38, 40]. In these studies, adherence to CONSORT 2010 Statement was explicitly mentioned. Several studies partially addressed these characteristics. Allocation concealment was missing in three studies [32, 37, 39], and allocation concealment and blinding were not addressed in another study [25]. Interestingly, CONSORT 2010 Statement was followed in these studies [25, 32, 39] indicating that the authors were aware of the checklist items. A recent RCT study only mentioned randomization but without clear explanation of the procedure, and did not report on sample size, allocation concealment and blinding [33]. A prospective clinical trial did not report on any of the four important study design features [15]. As expected, the latter two studies contain no reference to CONSORT 2010 Statement [15, 33]. Despite the fact that CONSORT 2010 Statement specifically addresses reporting of RCTs, authors of other types of clinical trials are encouraged to report their studies following CONSORT 2010 Statement [30].

Further progress in conducting clinical trials on bulk-fill composites is evidenced in increased use of rubber dam for moisture control. Rubber dam was reported in the majority of recent clinical trials with only a few using rubber dam selectively or entirely relying on cotton rolls and suction (Appendix 1, Table 9.1). This is unlike the finding of previously mentioned meta-analyses in which cotton rolls were found to be the main moisture control tool [23, 28]. Though this is a positive trend in conducting clinical trials, it may alienate clinical trials in university settings from general practice as the majority of dentists still opt not to use rubber dam for restorative procedures [44, 45] similar to the observations in general practice more than 10 years ago [46].

9.3.3 Clinical Challenges of Bulk-Fill Composites

Clinical challenges for bulk-fill composites are similar to composites in general. This is evidenced in the same main reasons for restoration failure: secondary caries, tooth and restoration fractures, post-operative sensitivity and inflammation, anatomical shape, marginal adaptation and discoloration and loss of retention.

Secondary caries was shown to be partly material dependent as it was significantly more associated with composite than amalgam [47, 48]. Technique sensitivity, no antimicrobial properties, affinity for bacterial growth and presence of gaps were identified as contributing factors to secondary caries related to composite restorations [47]. Gingival margins of Class II restorations are particularly vulnerable to secondary caries. In terms of patient's status, high caries risk and smoking were identified as significant contributing factors to secondary caries [48].

A variety of factors may contribute to secondary caries at gingival margins, such as improper moisture control, poor adhesive bonding to dentin, material adaptation and light-curing. The same challenges apply for bulk-fill composites, both sculptable and flowable, though the latter may not be associated so much with material adaptation as the former.

Rubber dam and proper moisture control is *condicio sine qua non* for proper composite polymerization which is, in turn, responsible for optimal material properties and ultimately clinical longevity. Various stakeholders, dental schools, manufacturers, insurance companies should put more effort in increased use of rubber dam in restorative dentistry. Patients should be better educated so they can develop and express expectation that their dentist uses rubber dam during restorative procedures.

Marginal adaptation may be improved with flowable materials. However, it is unknown whether flowable bulk-fill composites would be prone to defects in the area of proximal contacts similar to those found in glass ionomer restoratives [49, 50]. It is further unknown if these proximal defects occur due to material's chemical composition and/or inferior mechanical properties. It seems prudent that flowable composites are used for improved gingival adaptation but restricted to the area under proximal contacts and covered with sculptable universal or bulk-fill composites due to their generally better mechanical properties. Marginal adaptation of sculptable composites may be improved by material preheating [51]. A problem with preheated composites is that they cool down rapidly [52], so placement should occur as soon as the material is removed from the heater. Gap formation in the gingival margin in bulk-fill composites seems to be comparable to conventional composites [6]. Flowable bulk-fill composite SDR was found to induce smaller gap formation in dentin compared to sculptable materials [53]. It remains unclear if gap formation in bulk-fill composites contributes to secondary caries, but the risk seems no greater than that associated with conventional composites.

Adhesive bonding to dentin remains a challenge in contemporary adhesive dentistry and is not associated with composite material but rather with adhesive system, its composition, application mode and biodegradability. Current evidence supports three-step full etch-and-rinse (total-etch) approach and the preferred three-step combined selective enamel total-etch with two-self-etch bonding route for increased longevity of the adhesive-dentin bond [54].

Light-curing of bulk-fill composites should follow the same recommendations as for light-cured materials in general. Proper light-curing source and technique (diameter and positioning of the light tip and curing time) should ensure that sufficient energy is delivered to the material to maximize polymerization [55].

Tooth and restoration fracture risk should be addressed in the treatment planning phase. It is widely known that increased risk of tooth fracture is associated with insufficient cusp resistance, e.g. in endodontically treated teeth. Cuspal reduction of 2 mm and coverage with resin composite in MOD cavities of endodontically treated premolars and molars improves fracture resistance of such teeth [56, 57]. The remaining cavity wall thickness, even in the range of 1–1.5 mm does not seem to reduce significantly fracture resistance of teeth when proper cuspal protection is performed [58]. A clinical study on cusp-replacing complex composite restorations reported an annual failure rate of 0.9% over 96 months, the reasons for failure being endodontic complications, cusp fracture and inadequate proximal contact [59]. Composite materials with filler content above 74 vol% (compact composites [60]) may be suitable for complex composite restorations involving cusp replacement as their flexural modulus approaches 20 GPa which is expected for load-bearing restorations [61]. Sculptable bulk-fill composites do not exhibit such mechanical properties as compact composites [9, 62] and hence should not be used for complex composite restorations. Annual failure rates of Class I and II bulk-fill restorations in the available RCTs did not exceed the annual failure rate of composites in general [63] indicating that bulk-fill composites may be used for posterior restorations without cusp involvement.

Fiber-reinforced bulk-fill composite (introduced as Xenius, later rebranded as everX posterior, GC) is recommended for large cavity defects to replace dentin as a base material especially for high-stress bearing restorations [64]. In addition to the conventional filler particles in the BisGMA/TEGDMA-based resin matrix, this composite contains 1–2 mm glass fibers for improved fracture toughness and mechanical properties in general [65]. At 3 years, a somewhat lower clinical success rate was found for fiber-reinforced bulk-fill composite group (78.3%) compared to an incremental microhybrid composite restoration (91.3%) in endodontically treated molars of 24 patients, with fracture as the main reason for failure [66]. Another prospective clinical study following only the fiber-reinforced composite in posterior restoration in vital and non-vital molars and premolars reported an overall success rate of 88.9% for a period ranging from 1.3 to 4.3 years [67]. This is generally in line with findings for other composite materials, suggesting that fiber-reinforced bulk-fill may be a suitable base material for large cavities in posterior teeth.

Additionally, factor operator with regard to previous training and experience has not been investigated. It is unknown how the outcome of bulk-fill composite restorations might be influenced by the age of operator with older dentists trained in amalgam techniques. This challenge is not unique for bulk-fill composites, but for all innovations in dental practice. This highlights the importance of hands-on training and continuing professional development courses. The fact is that bulk-fill composites are applied to the cavity and sculpted in much the same way as universal composites, which have become materials of choice for posterior restorations and taken over amalgam. It is reasonable to expect that dentists primarily trained in amalgam techniques have already mastered universal composites over the course of their practice and that including bulk-fill composites in their everyday work should not present a challenge.

Appendix 2 shows clinical cases of teeth restored with different types of bulk-fill composites and followed at various periods of time ranging from 3 to 10 years. The restorations were placed by the same operator (JS) using different adhesive systems and illustrate the different failures reported in the literature such as secondary caries, fracture of the restoration, wear of composite and loss of esthetics, in general for composite materials [68] as well as for bulk-fill composites in this chapter.

As stated earlier, similar clinical performance in terms of esthetic, functional and biological FDI criteria was reported for bulk-fill composites as for conventional microhybrid composites. Failures occur at different periods of time, short term (1–3 years), medium term (3–6 years) and long term (6 years and above) (Appendix 1, Table 9.1). Management of those failures depends on the type of defect or problem, and can include monitoring, repair or total replacement of the restoration [69].

The clinical evaluation of bulk-fill composites (sculptable, flowable or fiber-reinforced) in Appendix 2 followed the same criteria as mentioned earlier in this chapter—FDI criteria set out in Hickel et al. [25] Evaluation of flowable and fiber-reinforced bulk-fill composites is only possible through radiography that may reveal some imperfections, voids or secondary caries.

9.3.4 Challenges in Clinical Evaluation of Bulk-Fill Composites

The main challenges in clinical evaluation of bulk-fill composites are no different from other restorative dental materials. Dental research community still has not adequately responded to these challenges.

University vs. general practice setting—The majority of clinical trials are conducted in university settings with one or a few operators involved. In the reviewed clinical trials on bulk-fill composites, the number of operators did not exceed five

[35, 40] with the majority of trials involving only one operator [16, 17, 20, 21, 25, 31, 33, 37, 39]. The conditions are more strictly controlled with relatively narrow inclusion criteria in university clinical settings compared to general practice. This inevitably means that results from such clinical trials may not necessarily reflect a material's true performance in general practice.

Practice-based dental research (PBRNs) is not a new concept in dentistry and is considered to be a "real world" setting [70]. Dental PBRNs involve mostly private practitioners willing to conduct research within their practice. The main objective of this approach is to increase knowledge base for clinical decision-making by testing clinical approaches and effectiveness of strategies for the prevention, management and treatment of oral diseases and conditions [70]. A recent scoping review identified 24 dental PBRNs worldwide, from USA and Canada to Europe to Japan, Australia and New Zealand [71]. Material testing, clinical and in vitro, is the sole focus of the oldest PBRN, found in 1976, the CRA (Clinical Research Associates). However, dental restorative materials are included in many research projects by various networks. The National Dental Practice-Based Research Network, the largest PBRN in the world, involved 226 practitioners in evaluating 6218 direct composite and amalgam restorations in 3855 patients over 2 years [72]. The failure rate was 6.2% with no difference between material types, but with higher incidence of failures in patients over 65 years of age, in large restorations, in female clinicians and those practicing part-time. Among the most frequent reasons for failure were recurrent caries, loss of retention, tooth fracture, however the most frequent reason was found to be a repair/replacement of a restoration by another dentist [72].

A large retrospective PBRN-based study compared the longevity of nearly 360.000 composite, amalgam, glass ionomer and compomer restorations in more than 75.000 patients placed by 67 general dental practitioners [63]. The mean annual failure was 4.6% over 10 years, with the annual failure rate being 4.4% for composites, 5.1% for amalgam, 7.5% for compomer and 11.1% for glass ionomer cement restorations. Generally, the annual failure rate was found to increase in patients over 65 years of age (6.9%), in large 4+ surface restorations (6.0%), in molars (5.2%) and, especially, endodontically treated teeth (11.0%) [63]. Greater annual failure rate was reported for Class II than Class I restorations involving bulk-fill composite, 1.4% and 0% at 6 years, respectively [14], which is in line with findings for composite restorations in general [63, 72].

Only one study involving a bulk-fill composite in a PBRN setting was found in the literature [73]. In this study, a group of 12 dentists was asked to evaluate a sculptable bulk-fill composite in their practice. Handling of the material was found to be similar to composites previously used by the dentists, but its esthetic appearance was less favorably accepted. Despite the lack of PBRN-based clinical trials on the performance of bulk-fill composites, it is reasonable to expect similar results as for composites in general. This assumption is based on the findings from clinical trials in university settings which show similar clinical performance of bulk-fill and conventional incremental composites.

There is obvious strength in large numbers analysis, which is not possible to achieve in university-based clinical trials in a similar time frame, if ever. Yet, PBRNs have a number of limitations such as evaluator calibration [70], unbalanced test groups (multiple confounding factors) [72], inconsistencies in treatment protocol [74] and decision-making [75], operator- and practice-related differences (experience, skills, workload, practice size, location, type) [63, 72, 74], drop-out of practitioners throughout a trial [72]. One way of addressing limitations of PBRN-based clinical trials is implementing RCT study design. This would reduce the number of patients involved in such trials but would allow better control of variables and ultimately more meaningful results. Additionally, high quality calibration material and rigorous evaluator calibration would increase consistency and improve validity of results.

Low recall rate in long-term studies—A significant negative correlation was observed between the recall rate and observation period, suggesting the longer the trial, the lower the recall rate [76]. The same finding was seen in recently reported randomized clinical trials (RCTs) on bulk-fill composites [16, 21, 27] albeit there are examples of high recall rates [14]. Patient relocation, unavailability for contact and loss of interest in participating in the study were cited as the reasons for drop-out [16, 21]. Although the same decreasing trend can be found in PBRN-based studies [77], patients in private practices may be more inclined to be regular attendees of the same practice and attend regular follow-ups [63, 74] resulting in higher recall rates compared to university settings. Increase in PBRN-based research in general, proper selection of participating practices, data-sharing between different geographical locations and increased patient awareness of benefits in participating in clinical trials may improve recall rates in long-term clinical trials.

Low participant numbers—As seen in meta-analyses and recent RCTs, the number of patients per group remains below 50 in most cases. The number of participants per group is determined so that there is a high probability (at least 0.8), also known as "power," to detect a statistically significant difference between the study and control group based on the expected effect size between the test groups. The expected effect size or difference between the test groups can be estimated from published data, pilot trials or empirically. The problem with sample size calculation is this expected effect difference between the test groups. The true expected difference between groups may be rather small that it requires a large number of participants (large sample size). A large number of participants may be difficult to enrol in a university-based clinical trial with one or few operators performing the treatment. Conversely, participant numbers feasible for a university-based study may prove to be sufficient only to detect as statistically significant an unrealistically large difference between the test groups which makes the study not worth performing. A consequence of low participant numbers is that a difference between groups may be found not significant even though there may be clinical relevance in it. As university-based clinical trials struggle with sample size, this is a not an issue in PBRN-based studies. Moreover, pooling of restorations is a common practice in university-based studies, e.g. Class I and Class II or premolar and molar teeth, for statistical analysis. Tooth type, cavity size and the number of involved surfaces are significant factors determining the restoration annual failure rate [63, 72]. Unbalanced groups in this respect may affect statistical analysis.

Insufficient number of clinical trials—It is often stated that more clinical research on the performance of dental materials, especially newly launched materials, is required. The same is true for bulk-fill composites and recent meta-analyses clearly express the need for more, especially long-term, clinical trials [1, 23, 28]. This is true for clinical research in general, but more importantly for properly designed, conducted and reported RCTs. Short-term studies often cannot detect differences between bulk-fill and conventional composites as it may take long time for these differences to develop. Moreover, evaluation criteria, especially modified USPHS may be rather insensitive to slight differences in materials' performance.

Clinical trials in restorative dentistry are demanding in design and execution, take long time, have a number of confounding factors and progressively higher drop-outs and rely on subjective evaluators' assessment. Despite all efforts, it is difficult or impossible to overcome these limitations. Confounding factors, low recall rate and evaluators' subjectivity may be mitigated at best. Both university- and PBRN-based trials have their strengths and weaknesses. Both approaches are required to reach balance and improve the validity of findings to a degree that can strongly affect clinical practice.

9.4 Conclusions

Bulk-fill composites have shown similar clinical performance to conventional incremental composites in clinical trials. Restoration survival and annual failure rates are similar to conventional incremental composites. The main reason for restoration failure is secondary caries. Occasional differences in individual characteristics do not affect their overall clinically acceptable performance. Sculptable bulk-fill composites reduce restoration time, but the same has not been confirmed for flowable bulk-fill materials, likely due to the required capping layer of a sculptable composite. Clinical performance of bulk-fill composites is not influenced by the placement technique, adhesive system or technique and lining material. Challenges in clinical placement of bulk-fill composites are the same as for composites in general and include moisture control, proper adhesive placement technique, material adaptation and light-curing. Caution should be taken when restoring large cavities, especially in molar teeth. There is no clinical evidence to support the use of sculptable bulk-fill composites for cusp replacement in complex restorations and in vitro studies indicate their inferior mechanical properties for this indication. More well-designed, conducted and reported long-term randomized control trials are required to further elucidate clinical performance of bulk-fill composites. Conducting randomized clinical trials in practice-based network settings allows greater participant numbers, ability to detect smaller differences between test groups and better "real-life" research context.

Acknowledgments The author would like to express sincere gratitude to Professor Joseph Sabbagh for his clinical cases presented in Appendix 2 to illustrate clinical longevity of bulk-fill composites. The author is grateful to Professor Joseph Sabbagh and Professor Robert McConnell for their critical review of this chapter.

Appendix 1

Table 9.1 summarizes the main characteristics of clinical trials that were not included in recent meta-analyses for not meeting the inclusion criteria or for being published at later dates

Authors	Year	Type of study	Setting	Groups	Np-Nr (per group)	Follow-up	Class/ tooth type	Evaluation criteria	Rubber dam	Intervention group	Control group	Observation
Torres et al. [35]	2021	RCT split-mouth double blind	University 5 operators	Ormocer vs bulk-fill ormocer	30–30	2 years	Class II/ molar	FDI	Yes	Futurabond U (self-etch mode) + Admira fusion xtra	Futurabond U (self-etch mode) + Admira fusion	No sig. differences. Bulk-fill material required significantly shorter chair time
Hardan et al. [33]	2021	RCT split-mouth	University 1 operator	Bulk-fill vs incremental	30–30	12 months	Class I/ premolar and molar	Reduced FDI	Yes	Adper SingleBond (2-step total-etch) + Filtek bulk fill posterior	Adper SingleBond (totat-etch) + Filtek Z250XT	Initially no post-op pain in both groups, lower pain and marginal discolor-ation in bulk at 12 month than incremental. No caries
Cieplik et al. [32]	2021	RCT split-mouth blinded examiners	University 3 operators	SABF vs. sculptable bulk-fill	30–30	12 months	Class II/ premolar and molar	FDI	If possible	No adhesive, light cured 20s	ScotchBond universal (self-etch mode) + Filtek bulk fill one	All clinically acceptable scores; BF sign. better surface luster, marginal staining, color match than SABF, no diff. in other scores
Suneelku-mar et al. [39]	2021	RCT split-mouth double blind	University 1 operator	Bulk-fill incremental vs. bulk technique	42–42	12 months	Class I/ unstated	FDI	Yes	Single bond universal (self-etch mode) + Filtek bulk fill posterior, bulk technique	Single bond universal (self-etch mode) + Filtek bulk fill posterior, incremental technique	All restorations "excellent" or "clinically good" FDI scores. No sig. differences between two techniques

Yazici et al. [21]	**2021**	**RCT split-mouth double blind**	**University 1 operator**	**Bulk-fill vs. incremental composite**	**50–50**	**6 years**	**Class II/ premolar and molar**	**Modified USPHS**	**Yes**	**Excite (total-etch) + Tetric Evoceram bulk fill (TEC BF)**	**Adper single bond (total-etch) + Filtek ultimate (FU)**	**Sig. lower marginal discoloration for TEC BF than FU. Other criteria no sig. diff. Sig. worse marginal discoloration of FU than at baseline. Both sig. worse marginal adaptation than at baseline. No failure due to caries at 6 years**
Durão et al. [16]	**2021**	**RCT split-mouth double blind**	**University 1 operator**	**2 bulk-fill vs 1 incremental composite**	**46–46**	**3 years**	**Class I and II/ molar and premolar**	**Modified USPHS and FDI**	**Yes**	**1. Clearfil SE bond (selective-etch mode) + Tetric Evoceram bulk fill (TEC BF); 2. Clearfil SE bond (selective-etch mode) + Filtek bulk fill (FBF)**	**Clearfil SE bond (selective-etch mode) + Filtek Z250**	**TEC BF sig better surface luster than FBF and Z250 at 3 years. high-viscosity bulk-fill composites comparable to conventional incremental composite in a high caries incidence population. Sig. diff. Between USPHS and FDI criteria (surface roughness, marginal adaptation and staining). FDI more “success” scores, USPHS most “acceptable” scores**

(continued)

Table 9.1 (continued)

Authors	Year	Type of study	Setting	Groups	Np-Nr (per group)	Follow-up	Class/ tooth type	Evaluation criteria	Rubber dam	Intervention group	Control group	Observation
Torres et al. [40]	2020	RCT split-mouth double blind	University 5 operators	Bulk-fill composite with/without liner	30–30	2 years	Class I and II/molar and premolar	FDI	Yes	Ionoseal liner + Futurabond U (self-etch mode) + Admira fusion xtra	Futurabond U (self-etch mode) + Admira fusion xtra	No clinically "unsatisfactory" scores. No sig. diff. in criteria between two groups. 1 restoration per group "satisfactory" color match; 4 (liner) vs. 3 (no-liner) "satisfactory" marginal adaptation
Castro et al. [36]	2020	RCT split-mouth double blind	University 3 operators	Wet vs. dry bonding technique of a 2-step TE adhesive and 1 bulk-fill composite	45–45	12 months	Class I and II/molar and premolar	Reduced FDI	Yes	Wet-bonding Adper single Bond2 (total-etch) + Filtek bulk fill posterior	Dry-bonding Adper single Bond2 (total-etch) + Filtek bulk fill posterior	Ni sig. diff. in post-op sensitivity between groups. A sig. higher risk up to 48 h in both groups. No sig. diff. in marginal discoloration and adaptation, fracture and secondary caries. No effect of cavity type, depth or number of restored surfaces
ElAziz et al. [17]	**2020**	**RCT parallel blinded examiners**	**University 1 operator**	**Direct everX vs indirect onlays in complex restorations**	**38–38**	**12 months**	**Class II complex/ molars**	**Modified USPHS**	**Yes**	**Gaenial bond (selective-etch) + everX posterior + Gaenial posterior**	**Immediate dentin sealing (Futurabond 2-step self-etch) + dual cure adhesive cement (BifixQM) + GrandioSO**	**Marginal integrity of everX group sig. better than onlay. Color match sig. better in onlay group. No sig. diff. in other criteria**

Afifi et al [31]	**2019**	**RCT split mouth and parallel double blind**	**University 1 operator**	**Post-op sensitivity 1 month**	**30–15**	**1 months**	**Class II/ premolar and molar**	**VAS**	**No (cotton rolls + suction)**	**1. Total-etch adhesive (unspecified) + Tetric EvoCeram bulk fill; 2. Self-etch adhesive (unspecified) + Tetric EvoCeram bulk fill**	**1. Total-etch adhesive (unspecified) + Tetric EvoCeram; 2. Self-etch adhesive (unspecified) + Tetric EvoCeram**	**No sig. diff between the groups. Low sample size. Post-op sensitivity in bulk-fill initially and 1 week (total-etch), conventional occurred at 1 month (total-etch)**
Tardem et al. [34]	**2019**	**RCT split mouth double blind**	**University 4 operators**	**Self-etch vs. selective etch & bulk-fill vs. incremental**	**81–49 restorations**	**1 week**	**Class I and II/ premolar and molar**	**Numerical rating scale (NRT) and visual analog scale (VAS)**	**Yes**	**1. ScotchBond universal (SBU selective-etch) + Filtek one bulk fill (F1BF); 2. SBU (self-etch) + F1BF; 3. SBU (selective-etch) + FBF posterior; 4. SBU (self-etch) + FBF posterior**	**1. ScotchBond universal (selective-etch) + Filtek supreme ultra; 2. ScotchBond universal (self-etch) + Filtek supreme ultra**	**Twelve restorations in 6 patients post-op sensitivity (mild-moderate) to mastication/ air up to 48 h. overall risk of post-op sensitivity was 4%. Deeper cavities than 4 mm sig. more post-op sensitivity than shallower. Bulk-fills less time-consuming than incremental**
Fahim et al. [37]	2019	RCT, examiners blinded	University 1 operator	High-intensity vs. conventional LED (1 bulk-fill)	36 patients and 44 restorations in total	12 months	Class II/ premolar and molar	Modified USPHS	Yes	Futurabond U (selective-etch) + x-traFill (high-intensity 1400 mW/cm2 for 5 s)	Futurabond U (selective-etch) + x-traFill (low-intensity 650 mW/cm2 for 20s)	No sig. diff in criteria between groups. Significant increase in the % of marginal discontinuity of occlusal margins (impressions, SEM) at 12 m, more in "high-intensity" than "control" group

(continued)

Table 9.1 (continued)

Authors	Year	Type of study	Setting	Groups	Np-Nr (per group)	Follow-up	Class/ tooth type	Evaluation criteria	Rubber dam	Intervention group	Control group	Observation
Loguercio et al. [38]	2019	RCT split-mouth double blind	University 4 operators	Bulk-fill composite placed incrementally vs. bulk AND in total-etch vs self-etch adhesive	59–59	3 years	Class I and II/ premolar and molar	FDI	Yes	1. Tetric N-bond (total-etch) + Tetric EvoCeram bulk fill (as bulk); 2. Tetric N-bond SE (self-etch) + Tetric EvoCeram bulk fill (as bulk)	1. Tetric N-bond (total-etch) + Tetric EvoCeram bulk fill (as increm.); 2. Tetric N-bond SE (self-etch) + Tetric EvoCeram bulk fill (as increm.)	All restorations "acceptable" at 3 years. no caries after 3 years. 48 restorations (10–14 per group) immediate post-op sensitivity, no sig diff between groups. Marginal staining and adaptation sig worse in self-etch groups. No sig diff in other criteria
Akalın et al. [15]	*2018*	*Prospective clinical trial*	*University 2 operators*	*1 bulk-fill Sonicfill*	*52 patients in total, 111 restorations*	*2 years*	*Class II/ premolar and molar*	*Modified USPHS*	*No (cotton rolls + suction)*	*ScotchBond universal (selective-etch) + Sonic-Fill NB:2%CHX applied after rinsing the acid and before adhesive. Rubbed in for 10s, left for 10s and air-dried.*	*/*	*1 failure due to periapical inflammation, required RCT. Survival rate 99.1%. All received "acceptable" scores for color match, marginal staining and adaptation, anatomic form, surface roughness. Post-op sensitivity 0 at baseline, but 2 at 2 years recall. No secondary caries. Color match, marginal discoloration and surface roughness start to deteriorate within 6 m*

Hickey et al. [43]	**2016**	**RCT parallel**	**General dental practice 1 operator**	**Bulk fill vs. incremental post-op sensitivity**	**72–36**	**2–30days**	**Class I and II/ premolar and molar**	**Question-naire**	**Yes**	**ScotchBond NT (total-etch) + SDR + Filtek Z250**	**ScotchBond NT (total-etch) + Filtek Z250**	**At day 2, 18 (25%) teeth-postop pain, sig more in SDR group. At day, 7 *(11%) teeth- postop pain, no diff between groups. At day 30, 2 (3%) teeth-postop pain. Not unclear whether pain was spontaneous/cold/air. More class I tender to biting than class II**
Sarret et al. [20]	*2006*	*Prospec-tive clinical trial*	*University 1 operator*	*Bulk-fill*	*32 patient, 57 restora-tions*	*3 years*	*Class II/ premolar and molar*	*Modified USPHS*	*Yes*	*OptiBond solo (total-etch) + prodigy*	/	*<50% recall rate. Clinically unacceptable score requiring replacement 8% marginal adaptation and proximal contact, 4% caries, anatomical form and retention*

References in **Bold**—RCTs with Conventional Composite as Control; References in Normal Font—RCTs with Bulk-Fill in both Test Groups with Control Related to, e.g., Bonding, Placement Technique, Lining, Light-Curing; References in *Italic*—Prospective Clinical Trials with no Control Group

Appendix 2: Clinical Examples

Case 1

A class II SDR and Ceramex restoration at 8.5 years, the restoration is considered "clinically unsatisfactory but repairable" (too weak (open) contact, 100 micron metal blade can pass, inadequate proximal contour and potential soft tissue damage due to food impaction). The space between the molar and the premolar is due to a generalized periodontal problem. The radiography shows no secondary caries, a perfect adaptation of the composite on the cavity walls and a porosity in the middle of the restoration which indicates an air-bubble trapped during injection of flowable composite (Fig. 9.2).

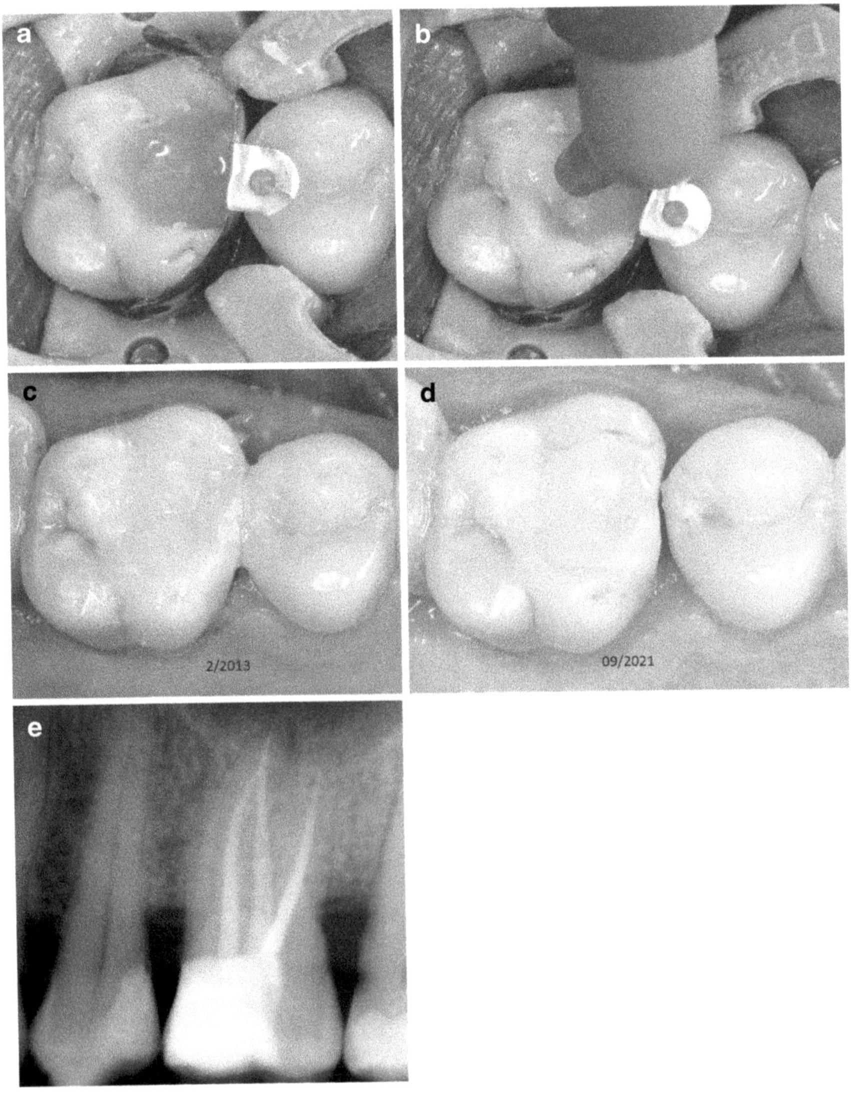

Fig. 9.2 SDR and Ceramex at 8 years

Case 2

The use of flowable bulk-fill composite Xtra Base (Voco) in a deep class I cavity, covered by Amaris (Voco).

At 5 years, the restoration is considered excellent/very good from a functional and esthetic point of view. The form is ideal and the luster similar to that of enamel. The radiography shows no pathology (secondary caries) and a harmonious transition between restoration and tooth (Fig. 9.3).

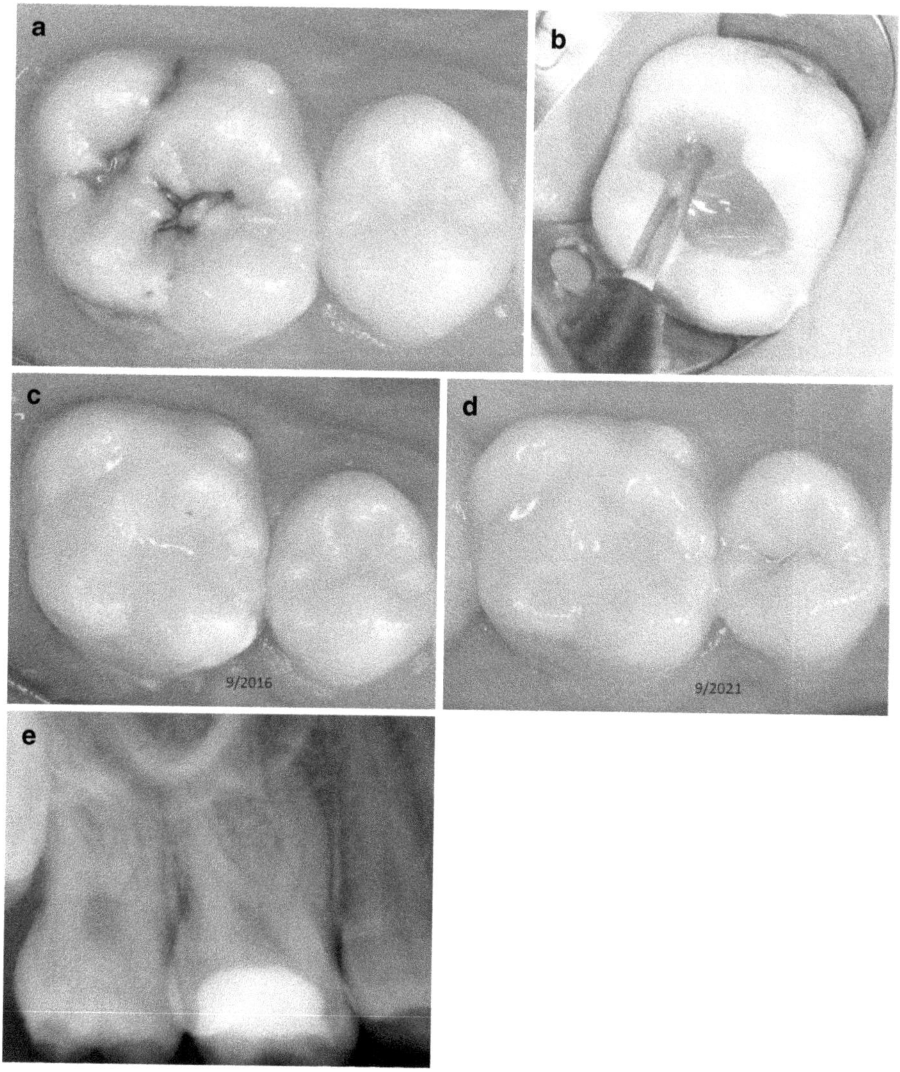

Fig. 9.3 Xtra Base + Amaris

Case 3

Restoration of a class II (OD) and a class I using Sonicfill 1, a sculptable and sonically activated bulk-fill resin composites with Optibond FL. At 9 years, the restorations show good marginal adaptation and anatomical shape but a loss of surface luster.

It is considered clinically sufficient/satisfactory from an esthetic point of view since the surface is dull but acceptable if covered with saliva film. From a functional point of view, it is considered clinically good with a slight visible margin on the lingual cusp of the first molar (Fig. 9.4).

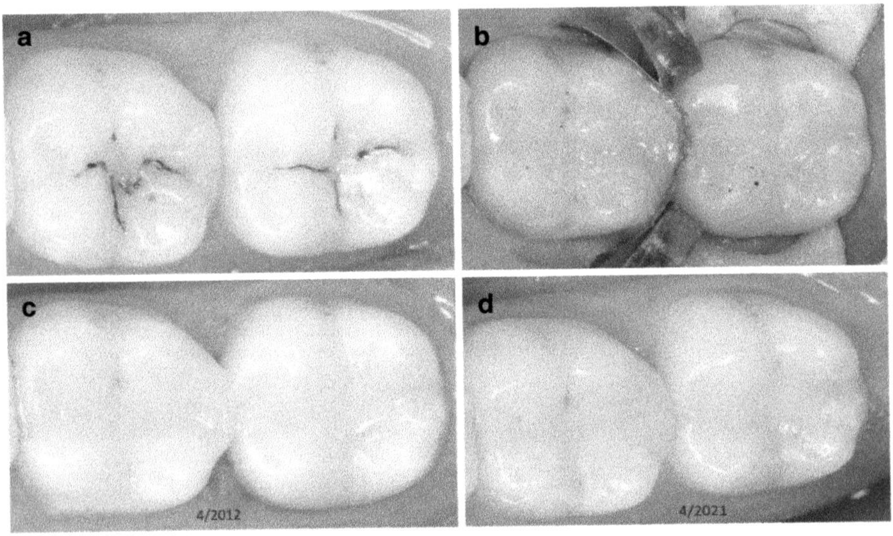

Fig. 9.4 Sonicfill restoration

Case 4

Restoration of a class II (OM) using Sonicfill 1, a sculptable and sonically activated bulk-fill resin composites with Optibond XTR. At 8 years, the restoration shows severe wear and loss of anatomical shape and surface luster. It is considered clinically sufficient/satisfactory from a functional and esthetic point of view with gaps <250 μm (Fig. 9.5).

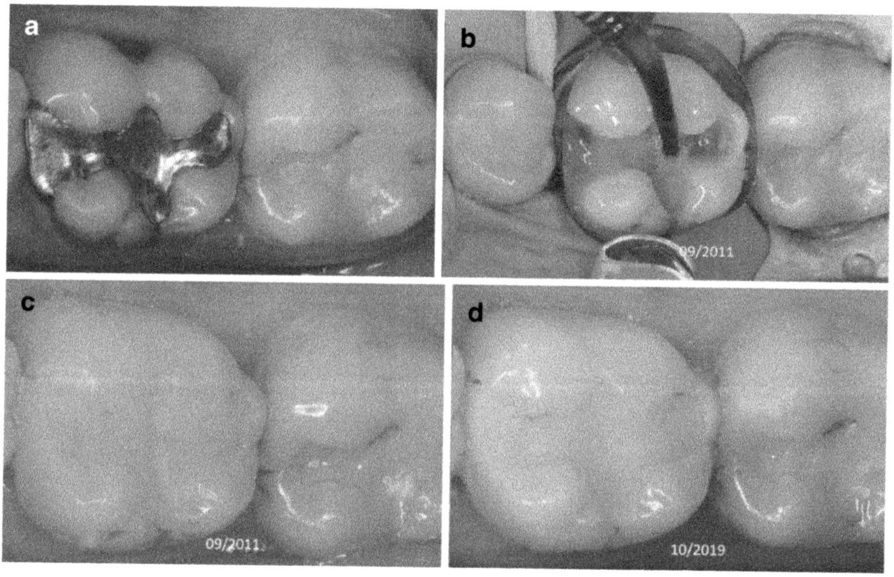

Fig. 9.5 Sonicfill 1 + Optibond XTR

Case 5

Sonicfill 1 at 9 years shows marginal fracture and secondary caries (tooth 46), and moderate surface staining 9 (tooth 48)—clinically sufficient/satisfactory (Fig. 9.6).

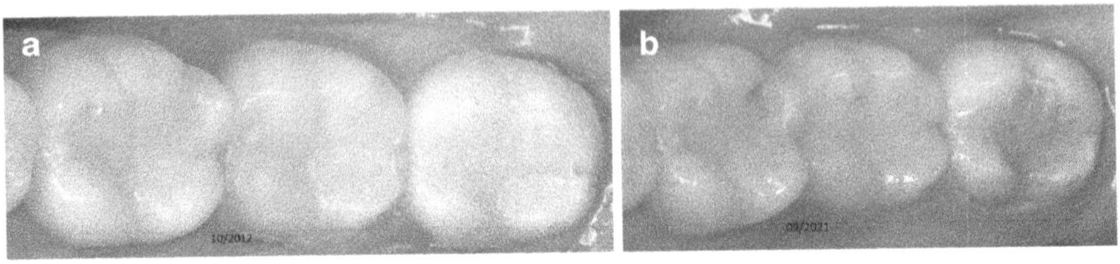

Fig. 9.6 Sonicfill Three class I cavities

Case 6

At 8 years, a class II Sonicfill restoration shows caries and cavitation and is considered "clinically unsatisfactory/poor" and too weak contact point with food impaction and requires replacement (Fig. 9.7).

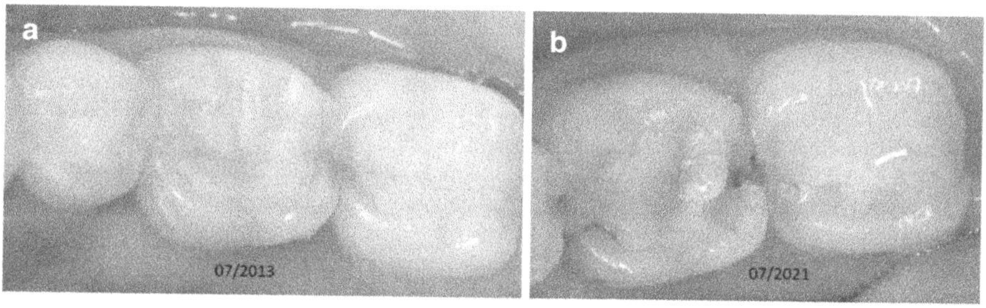

Fig. 9.7 Sonicfill: Secondary caries and fracture at 8 years

References

1. Cidreira Boaro LC, Pereira Lopes D, de Souza ASC, et al. Clinical performance and chemical-physical properties of bulk fill composites resin -a systematic review and meta-analysis. Dent Mater. 2019;35:e249–64.
2. Miletic V, Pongprueksa P, De Munck J, Brooks NR, Van Meerbeek B. Curing characteristics of flowable and sculptable bulk-fill composites. Clin Oral Investig. 2017;21:1201–12.
3. Ilie N, Kessler A, Durner J. Influence of various irradiation processes on the mechanical properties and polymerisation kinetics of bulk-fill resin based composites. J Dent. 2013;41:695–702.
4. Ilie N, Bucuta S, Draenert M. Bulk-fill resin-based composites: an in vitro assessment of their mechanical performance. Oper Dent. 2013;38:618–25.
5. Alshali RZ, Salim NA, Satterthwaite JD, Silikas N. Post-irradiation hardness development, chemical softening, and thermal stability of bulk-fill and conventional resin-composites. J Dent. 2015;43:209–18.
6. El Naga MA, Qian F, Denehy GE, Quock RL, Armstrong SR. Marginal adaptation and internal indentation resistance of a class II bulk-fill resin-based composite. Am J Dent. 2020;33:145–50.
7. Benetti AR, Havndrup-Pedersen C, Honore D, Pedersen MK, Pallesen U. Bulk-fill resin composites: polymerization contraction, depth of cure, and gap formation. Oper Dent. 2015;40:190–200.
8. Campos EA, Ardu S, Lefever D, Jasse FF, Bortolotto T, Krejci I. Marginal adaptation of class II cavities restored with bulk-fill composites. J Dent. 2014;42:575–81.
9. Leprince JG, Palin WM, Vanacker J, Sabbagh J, Devaux J, Leloup G. Physico-mechanical characteristics of commercially available bulk-fill composites. J Dent. 2014;42:993–1000.
10. Bellinaso MD, Soares FZM, Rocha RO. Do bulk-fill resins decrease the restorative time in posterior teeth? A systematic review and meta-analysis of in vitro studies. J Investig Clin Dent. 2019;10:e12463.
11. Cvar JF, Ryge G. Reprint of criteria for the clinical evaluation of dental restorative materials. 1971. Clin Oral Investig. 2005;9:215–32.
12. Bayne SC, Schmalz G. Reprinting the classic article on USPHS evaluation methods for measuring the clinical research performance of restorative materials. Clin Oral Investig. 2005;9:209–14.
13. van Dijken JW, Pallesen U. Posterior bulk-filled resin composite restorations: a 5-year randomized controlled clinical study. J Dent. 2016;51:29–35.
14. van Dijken JWV, Pallesen U. Bulk-filled posterior resin restorations based on stress-decreasing resin technology: a randomized, controlled 6-year evaluation. Eur J Oral Sci. 2017;125:303–9.
15. Akaliotan TT, Bozkurt FO, Kusdemir M, Ozsoy A, Ozcan M. Clinical evaluation of sonic-activated high viscosity bulk-fill Nanohybrid resin composite restorations in class II cavities: a prospective clinical study up to 2 years. Eur J Prosthodont Restor Dent. 2018;26:152–60.
16. Durao MA, de Andrade AKM, do Prado AM, et al. Thirty-six-month clinical evaluation of posterior high-viscosity bulk-fill resin composite restorations in a high caries incidence population: interim results of a randomized clinical trial. Clin Oral Investig. 2021;25(11):6219–37.
17. ElAziz RH, Mohammed MM, Gomaa HA. Clinical performance of short-fiber-reinforced resin composite restorations vs resin composite onlay restorations in complex cavities of molars (randomized clinical trial). J Contemp Dent Pract. 2020;21:296–303.
18. Balkaya H, Arslan S, Pala K. A randomized, prospective clinical study evaluating effectiveness of a bulk-fill composite resin, a conventional composite resin and a reinforced glass ionomer in class II cavities: one-year results. J Appl Oral Sci. 2019;27:e20180678.
19. Frascino S, Fagundes TC, Silva U, et al. Randomized prospective clinical trial of class II restorations using low-shrinkage flowable resin composite. Oper Dent. 2020;45:19–29.
20. Sarrett DC, Brooks CN, Rose JT. Clinical performance evaluation of a packable posterior composite in bulk-cured restorations. J Am Dent Assoc. 2006;137:71–80.
21. Yazici AR, Kutuk ZB, Ergin E, Karahan S, Antonson SA. Six-year clinical evaluation of bulk-fill and nanofill resin composite restorations. Clin Oral Investig. 2021;26(1):417–26.

22. Guney T, Yazici AR. 24-month clinical evaluation of different bulk-fill restorative resins in class II restorations. Oper Dent. 2020;45:123–33.
23. Veloso SRM, Lemos CAA, de Moraes SLD, do Egito Vasconcelos BC, Pellizzer EP, de Melo Monteiro GQ. Clinical performance of bulk-fill and conventional resin composite restorations in posterior teeth: a systematic review and meta-analysis. Clin Oral Investig. 2019;23:221–33.
24. Hickel R, Roulet JF, Bayne S, et al. Recommendations for conducting controlled clinical studies of dental restorative materials. Science Committee Project 2/98—FDI World Dental Federation study design (Part I) and criteria for evaluation (Part II) of direct and indirect restorations including onlays and partial crowns. J Adhes Dent. 2007;9(Suppl 1):121–47.
25. Hickel R, Peschke A, Tyas M, et al. FDI world dental federation—clinical criteria for the evaluation of direct and indirect restorations. Update and clinical examples. J Adhes Dent. 2010;12:259–72.
26. Manhart J, Chen HY, Hickel R. Three-year results of a randomized controlled clinical trial of the posterior composite QuiXfil in class I and II cavities. Clin Oral Investig. 2009;13:301–7.
27. Heck K, Manhart J, Hickel R, Diegritz C. Clinical evaluation of the bulk fill composite QuiXfil in molar class I and II cavities: 10-year results of a RCT. Dent Mater. 2018;34:e138–47.
28. Arbildo-Vega HI, Lapinska B, Panda S, Lamas-Lara C, Khan AS, Lukomska-Szymanska M. Clinical effectiveness of bulk-fill and conventional resin composite restorations: systematic review and meta-analysis. Polymers (Basel). 2020;12:12.
29. Kruly PC, Giannini M, Pascotto RC, et al. Meta-analysis of the clinical behavior of posterior direct resin restorations: low polymerization shrinkage resin in comparison to methacrylate composite resin. PLoS One. 2018;13:e0191942.
30. Schulz KF, Altman DG, Moher D, Group C. CONSORT 2010 statement: updated guidelines for reporting parallel group randomised trials. BMJ. 2010;340:c332.
31. Afifi SMH, Haridy MF, Farid MR. Evaluation of post-operative sensitivity of bulk fill resin composite versus Nano resin composite: a randomized controlled clinical study. Open Access Maced J Med Sci. 2019;7:2335–42.
32. Cieplik F, Scholz KJ, Anthony JC, et al. One-year results of a novel self-adhesive bulk-fill restorative and a conventional bulk-fill composite in class II cavities-a randomized clinical split-mouth study. Clin Oral Investig. 2022;26(1):449–61.
33. Hardan L, Sidawi L, Akhundov M, et al. One-year clinical performance of the fast-Modelling bulk technique and composite-up layering technique in class I cavities. Polymers. 2021;13:19.
34. Tardem C, Albuquerque EG, Lopes LS, et al. Clinical time and postoperative sensitivity after use of bulk-fill (syringe and capsule) vs. incremental filling composites: a randomized clinical trial. Braz Oral Res. 2019;33:e089.
35. Torres CR, Jurema AL, Souza MY, Di Nicolo R, Borges AB. Bulk-fill versus layering pure ormocer posterior restorations: a randomized split-mouth clinical trial. Am J Dent. 2021;34:143–9.
36. Castro AS, Maran BM, Gutierrez MF, et al. Dentin moisture does not influence postoperative sensitivity in posterior restorations: a double-blind randomized clinical trial. Am J Dent. 2020;33:206–12.
37. Fahim SE, Mostafa MA, Abi-Elhassan MH, Taher HM. Clinical behaviour and marginal sealing of bulk-fill resin composite restorations using light amplified high-intensity LEDs curing: a randomized controlled clinical trial. Open Access Maced J Med Sci. 2019;7:1360–8.
38. Loguercio AD, Rezende M, Gutierrez MF, Costa TF, Armas-Vega A, Reis A. Randomized 36-month follow-up of posterior bulk-filled resin composite restorations. J Dent. 2019;85:93–102.
39. Suneelkumar C, Harshala P, Madhusudhana K, Lavanya A, Subha A, Swapna S. Clinical performance of class I cavities restored with bulk fill composite at a 1-year follow-up using the FDI criteria: a randomized clinical trial. Restor Dent Endod. 2021;46:e24.
40. Torres CRG, Mailart MC, Rocha RS, et al. The influence of a liner on deep bulk-fill restorations: randomized clinical trial. J Dent. 2020;102:103454.
41. Durao MA, Andrade AKM, Santos M, Montes M, Monteiro GQM. Clinical performance of bulk-fill resin composite restorations using the United States Public Health Service and

federation dentaire internationale criteria: a 12-month randomized clinical trial. Eur J Dent. 2021;15:179–92.
42. Costa T, Rezende M, Sakamoto A, et al. Influence of adhesive type and placement technique on postoperative sensitivity in posterior composite restorations. Oper Dent. 2017;42:143–54.
43. Hickey D, Sharif O, Janjua F, Brunton PA. Bulk dentine replacement versus incrementally placed resin composite: a randomised controlled clinical trial. J Dent. 2016;46:18–22.
44. Loch C, Ratnayake J, Veerasamy A, Cathro P, Lee R, Brunton PA. Direct restorations, Endodontics, and bleaching: materials and techniques used by general dentists of New Zealand. Int J Dent. 2019;2019:6327171.
45. Wilson NHF, Burke FJT, Brunton PA, Creanor S, Hosey MT, Mannocci F. Dental practice in the UK in 2015/2016. Part 2: aspects of direct restorations, bleaching, endodontics and paediatric dentistry. Br Dent J. 2019.
46. Gilbert GH, Litaker MS, Pihlstrom DJ, Amundson CW, Gordan VV, Group DC. Rubber dam use during routine operative dentistry procedures: findings from the dental PBRN. Oper Dent. 2010;35:491–9.
47. Nedeljkovic I, Teughels W, De Munck J, Van Meerbeek B, Van Landuyt KL. Is secondary caries with composites a material-based problem? Dent Mater. 2015;31:e247–77.
48. Nedeljkovic I, De Munck J, Vanloy A, et al. Secondary caries: prevalence, characteristics, and approach. Clin Oral Investig. 2020;24:683–91.
49. Scholtanus JD, Huysmans MC. Clinical failure of class-II restorations of a highly viscous glass-ionomer material over a 6-year period: a retrospective study. J Dent. 2007;35:156–62.
50. Balkaya H, Arslan S. A two-year clinical comparison of three different restorative materials in class II cavities. Oper Dent. 2020;45:E32–42.
51. Lucey S, Lynch CD, Ray NJ, Burke FM, Hannigan A. Effect of pre-heating on the viscosity and microhardness of a resin composite. J Oral Rehabil. 2010;37:278–82.
52. Rueggeberg FA, Daronch M, Browning WD, MF DEG. In vivo temperature measurement: tooth preparation and restoration with preheated resin composite. J Esthet Restor Dent. 2010;22:314–22.
53. Peutzfeldt A, Mühlebach S, Lussi A, Flury S. Marginal gap formation in approximal "bulk fill" resin composite restorations after artificial ageing. Oper Dent. 2018;43:180–9.
54. Van Meerbeek B, Yoshihara K, Van Landuyt K, Yoshida Y, Peumans M. From Buonocore's pioneering acid-etch technique to self-adhering restoratives. A status perspective of rapidly advancing dental adhesive technology. J Adhes Dent. 2020;22:7–34.
55. Price R. In: Miletic V, editor. Dental composite materials for direct restorations. 1st ed. Cham: Springer International; 2018. p. 43–62.
56. Mondelli RF, Ishikiriama SK, de Oliveira FO, Mondelli J. Fracture resistance of weakened teeth restored with condensable resin with and without cusp coverage. J Appl Oral Sci. 2009;17:161–5.
57. Frankenberger R, Zeilinger I, Krech M, et al. Stability of endodontically treated teeth with differently invasive restorations: adhesive vs. non-adhesive cusp stabilization. Dent Mater. 2015;31:1312–20.
58. ElAyouti A, Serry MI, Geis-Gerstorfer J, Lost C. Influence of cusp coverage on the fracture resistance of premolars with endodontic access cavities. Int Endod J. 2011;44:543–9.
59. Scholtanus JD, Ozcan M. Clinical longevity of extensive direct composite restorations in amalgam replacement: up to 3.5 years follow-up. J Dent. 2014;42:1404–10.
60. Randolph LD, Palin WM, Leloup G, Leprince JG. Filler characteristics of modern dental resin composites and their influence on physico-mechanical properties. Dent Mater. 2016;32:1586–99.
61. Kinney JH, Marshall SJ, Marshall GW. The mechanical properties of human dentin: a critical review and re-evaluation of the dental literature. Crit Rev Oral Biol Med. 2003;14:13–29.
62. Shibasaki S, Takamizawa T, Nojiri K, et al. Polymerization behavior and mechanical properties of high-viscosity bulk fill and low shrinkage resin composites. Oper Dent. 2017;42:E177–87.

63. Laske M, Opdam NJ, Bronkhorst EM, Braspenning JC, Huysmans MC. Longevity of direct restorations in dutch dental practices. descriptive study out of a practice based research network. J Dent. 2016;46:12–7.
64. Garoushi S, Sailynoja E, Vallittu PK, Lassila L. Physical properties and depth of cure of a new short fiber reinforced composite. Dent Mater. 2013;29:835–41.
65. Garoushi S. In: Miletic M, editor. Dental composite materials for direct restorations. Cham: Springer International; 2018. p. 119–28.
66. Tekce N, Aydemir S, Demirci M, Tuncer S, Sancak EI, Baydemir C. Clinical performance of direct posterior composite restorations with and without short glass-fiber-reinforced composite in endodontically treated teeth: 3-year results. J Adhes Dent. 2020;22:127–37.
67. Tanner J, Tolvanen M, Garoushi S, Sailynoja E. Clinical evaluation of fiber-reinforced composite restorations in posterior teeth-results of 2.5 year follow-up. Open Dent J. 2018;12:476–85.
68. Moraes RR, Cenci MS, Scheneider LFJ. In: Miletic V, editor. Dental composite materials for direct restorations. Springer International: Cham; 2018. p. 269–88.
69. Hickel R, Brushaver K, Ilie N. Repair of restorations—criteria for decision making and clinical recommendations. Dent Mater. 2013;29:28–50.
70. Mjör IA. Practice-based dental research. J Oral Rehabil. 2007;34:913–20.
71. Canceill T, Monsarrat P, Faure-Clement E, Tohme M, Vergnes J-N, Grosgogeat B. Dental practice-based research networks (D-PBRN) worldwide: a scoping review. J Dent. 2021;104:103523.
72. McCracken MS, Gordan VV, Litaker MS, et al. A 24-month evaluation of amalgam and resin-based composite restorations: findings from the national dental practice-based research network. J Am Dent Assoc. 2013;144:583–93.
73. Burke FJT, Crisp RJ, Panchal D, Redfearn P, Sands P. A practice-based clinical evaluation of a bulk fill restorative material. Eur J Prosthodont Restor Dent. 2016;24:152–7.
74. Hilton TJ, Ferracane JL, Mancl L. Northwest practice-based research collaborative in evidence-based D. comparison of CaOH with MTA for direct pulp capping: a PBRN randomized clinical trial. J Dent Res. 2013;92:16S–22S.
75. Gordan VV, Riley J 3rd, Geraldeli S, Williams OD, Spoto JC 3rd, Gilbert GH. The decision to repair or replace a defective restoration is affected by who placed the original restoration: findings from the National dental PBRN. J Dent. 2014;42:1528–34.
76. Brunthaler A, Konig F, Lucas T, Sperr W, Schedle A. Longevity of direct resin composite restorations in posterior teeth. Clin Oral Investig. 2003;7:63–70.
77. Hilton TJ, Funkhouser E, Ferracane JL, et al. Baseline characteristics as 3-year predictors of tooth fracture and crack progression: findings from the national dental practice-based research network. J Am Dent Assoc. 2021;152:146–56.

Bulk-Fill Resin Composites: Recent Advances and Future Perspectives

10

Ahmad A. Jum'ah and Paul A. Brunton

10.1 Self-Adhesive Resin-Based Bulk-Fill Materials

Adhesive bonding of conventional direct resin composite restorations is a complex, technique sensitive, and time-consuming process. It requires application and curing of the adhesive resin layer prior to the placement of the resin composite. Self-adhesive restoratives would negate the need for tooth surface conditioning, adhesive bonding, and mechanical retentive features, where indicated. Self-adhesive materials are highly desired by clinicians owing to their efficiency and use for treating challenging situations such as uncooperative patients, cases where prolonged moisture control is unfeasible, or patients who cannot tolerate lengthy dental treatment due to chronic medical conditions.

The global trend of amalgam phasedown has driven significant research and development on self-adhering bulk-fill amalgam substitutes. Resin modified glass ionomer (RMGI) based restoratives are amongst the most widely used and tested materials. This group of materials exhibits the advantages of bulk-fill restoratives in addition to their cariostatic activity due to the fluoride release. However, reduced bonding to tooth structure [1], lack of strength [2] as well as their diminished wear resistance [2, 3], and moisture sensitivity [4] are among the major drawbacks of these materials.

A. A. Jum'ah (✉)
Restorative Dentistry Department, Faculty of Dentistry, Jordan University of Science and Technology, Irbid, Jordan

Faculty of Dentistry, Aqaba Medical Sciences University, Aqaba, Jordan
e-mail: aajuma@just.edu.jo

P. A. Brunton
Division of Health Sciences, University of Otago, Dunedin, New Zealand

Curtin University, Perth, Western Australia
e-mail: paul.brunton@curtin.edu.au

J. Sabbagh, R. McConnell (eds.), *Bulk Fill Resin Composites in Dentistry*,
https://doi.org/10.1007/978-3-031-16388-3_10

Conventional resin composites are inherently unable to bond to tooth structure and thereby an adhesive system should be used with such restorations [5]. That being said, several strategies have been implemented to produce self-adhering resin composites in order to simplify restorative treatments. One of the earliest strategies was to modify the viscosity controller monomers or the so-called reactive diluents. The modification involves addition of acidic moieties to the reactive diluents in order to promote adhesion to tooth structure. This group of materials bonds to tooth structure primarily via the interaction of phosphate functional groups with calcium ions within hydroxyapatite crystals and secondarily through micromechanical interlocking between the polymerized monomer and collagen fibres of dentin.

10.1.1 Self-Adhesive Resin Composites with Acidic Resin Matrix

One of the earliest commercially available self-adhering flowable composites (Vertise Flow; Kerr, CA, USA) contained a phosphoric-acid ester methacrylate and glycerol-phosphate dimethacrylate (GPDMA) as acidic functional monomers [1]. The phosphate functional group had an acidic phosphate group for etching tooth structure and two methacrylate groups for co-polymerization with other methacrylate monomers [6]. Despite the lower nano-leakage exhibited by such self-adhering flowable composites compared to conventional counterparts [5], its' retention and bond strength to dentin and interfacial adaptation to enamel and dentin have been sub-optimal as indicated by in vitro [6, 7] and clinical [8] studies. Fusio Liquid Dentin (Pentron, Orange, CA, USA), another commercially available self-adhering flowable resin composite that chemically bonds to tooth structure using 4-methacryloxyethyl trimellitic acid (4-META) which is able to partially demineralise dentin and to form ionic bonds between its carboxylate groups and calcium ions [9]. The latter material was associated with low bond strength [9, 10] and poor clinical performance [11]. One experimental self-adhesive, micro-hybrid resin composite material (code: Exp.564, 3 M Oral Care, Seefeld, Germany) was investigated [12]. The two-paste material utilized the well-known phosphoric acid-6-methacryloxy-hexylesters (15–25% wt) adhesive monomer [12]. Preliminary micro-tensile bond strength data suggested optimal bonding to dentin though less promising results were observed with enamel. Furthermore, interfacial analysis using transmission electron microscopy revealed a tight interface formed between the experimental material and bur-cut enamel and dentin with limited evidence of micro-tag formation and superficial demineralisation [12].

10.1.2 Modified Polyacid Systems (MOPOS)

Recently, a new self-adhesive bulk-fill resin composite was commercially introduced as Surefil One (SF-I; Dentsply Sirona, Germany). The self-adhesive properties of this material are obtained via modification of the structural monomer rather than the reactive diluent. The key component of this material is the patented modified polyacid system (MOPOS). The modification involves the use of polyacids, similar to those used in glass ionomer (GI) as a backbone. The high number of carboxylate groups within the polyacid backbone allows adhesion with enamel and dentin via ionic bonds with calcium ions within the tooth structure. Furthermore, acidic groups can bond the structural monomer to the glass fillers. The formation of an ionic bond between the carboxylate groups and calcium ions requires an aqueous environment, hence the addition of water to the formula of SF-I. The presence of water necessitates the use of hydrolytically stable, polymerizable groups (methacrylamide) that can be crosslinked with the reactive diluent. Furthermore, cross-linker molecules and reactive diluent need to be water-soluble and hydrolytically stable. In SF-I, a medium viscosity cross-linker with two polymerizable groups (BADEP) is used. A low viscosity reactive diluent, the acrylic acid, which also can adhere to tooth structure and reactive fillers via ionic bonds is also used in SF-I. Barium glass fillers of conventional resin composites cannot be used in SF-I owing to the presence of water in the formula. The low refractive index filler system used in SF-I contains aluminium-phosphor-strontium-sodium-fluorosilicate glass, highly dispersed silicon dioxide and ytterbium fluoride. Silanization of the fillers allows strong adhesion to the resin matrix within the system. The material is available in light-cure or self-cure modes. The light polymerization initiator system is comprised of camphorquinone along with two different reducing agents. To fulfil the bulk-fill objective, a redox initiator (potassium persulphate) is used to initiate radical polymerization reaction in order to mediate the chemical or dark cure process of SF-I. Figure 10.1: Graphical illustration of various components of the SF-I and their interaction among each other and with tooth structure.

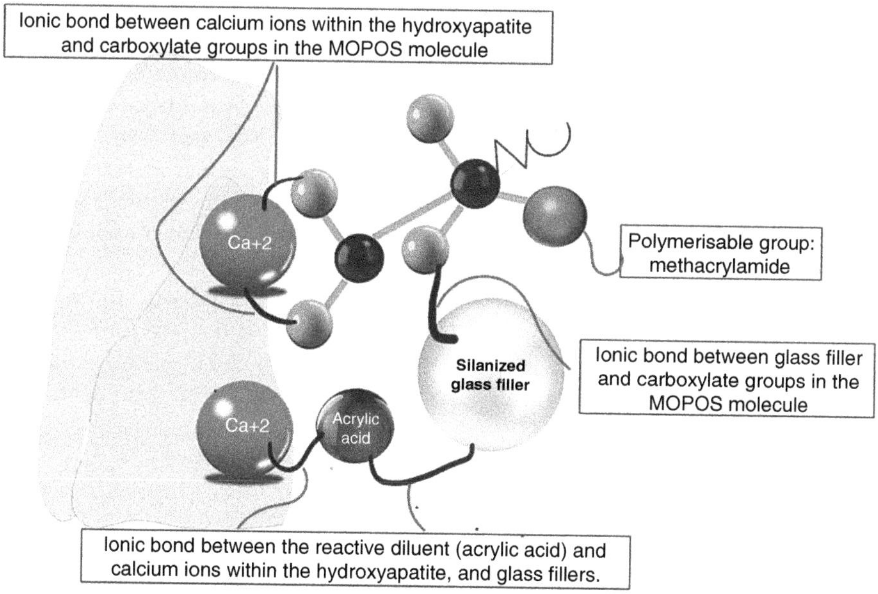

Fig. 10.1 The components of Surefill one

The evidence pertaining to the bonding effectiveness of SF-I to tooth structure is limited. Shear bond strength of SF-I to enamel was comparable to that obtained with a conventional resin composite bonded using a universal self-etch adhesive [13]. SF-I also exhibited similar bond strength to dentin when compared to a light cured RMGI or hybrid glass restorative materials. The bond strength of such materials was, however, significantly lower when compared to a conventional resin composite bonded with a universal, self-etch adhesive [13]. Nonetheless, shear bond strength values of SF-I (21–26 MPa) may be within clinically acceptable values and similar to materials with favourable long-term clinical success. Furthermore, the bond strength of SF-I to dentin was similar when the material is applied to moist or desiccated dentin indicating that using such material may reduce the incidence of post-operative sensitivity associated with excessive drying of dentin and may be more forgiving in cases where optimum moisture control cannot be achieved [14]. Additionally, finishing of cavity preparation appeared to be critical to the bond strength of SF-I as the shear bond strength to dentin was significantly reduced when SF-I was applied to dentin covered with a thick smear layer [14]. The effectiveness of bonding of SF-I to dentin has been demonstrated in both flat dentin (low c-factor) and class I cavity preparations (high c-factor). The light-cured SF-I exhibited significantly higher immediate and post-fatigue microtensile bond strength to flat dentin when compared to a reference RMGI material. In high c-factor configurations, self-cured SF-I exhibited microtensile bond strength comparable to a bonded restoration placed using a self-etch adhesive, resin-based bulk-fill restorative material [1]. With regard to material wear, SF-I exhibited less localized and generalized wear when compared to GI, RMGI, and bioactive RMGI materials [3]. SF-I also exhibited mechanical performance close to that for some commercially available micro-filled (Heliomolar; Ivoclar Vivadent, Germany) and nano-filled resin composites (CeramX mono+; Dentsply Sirona, Germany). Processing the material in either self-cure or light-cure mode led to superior mechanical performance over a GI based material (Fuji II LC; GC, Japan) but significantly inferior when compared to a conventional, nano-cluster filled resin composite (Filtek Supreme; 3 M Oral Care, USA) [15]. Furthermore, SF-I exhibited stable fracture behaviour and comparable marginal quality as compared to resin composite bonded with self-etch adhesive when used as bulk MOD restorations in molar teeth especially when used in light-cured modus [2].

Self-adhering bulk-fill restoratives would be a significant asset in clinical practice. However, they should be thoroughly verified in vitro and tested for long-term durability in vivo. Table 10.1 summarizes the composition and literature pertaining the performance of some commercially available self-adhesive resin-containing bulk-fill materials.

Table 10.1 Self-adhesive resin-based composites

Materials	Manufacturer	Chemical composition	Filler load	Research data
Vertise flow	Kerr	• Resin: GPDMA, HEMA, Bis-GMA • Fillers: Pre-polymerized particles, colloidal silica, zinc oxide, silanated barium glass, ytterbium fluoride	Not specified SDS only reports 5–10% ytterbium fluoride content	Sub-optimal retention, adaptation, and clinical performance [6–8]
Fusio dentin liquid	Pentron Clinica	• Resin: UDMA, TEGDMA, HEMA, 4-META • Fillers: nano-sized amorphous silica, silane treated barium glass • Photo curing system: camphorquinone	Not specified	Low dentin bond strength and poor clinical performance [9–11]
Surefil one	Dentsply Sirona	• Structural monomer: Modified poly-acid with hydrolytically stable (methacryl-amide) groups • Reactive diluent: Acrylic acid • Filler: Aluminium-phosphor-strontium-sodium- fluorosilicate glass, highly dispersed silicon dioxide, ytterbium fluoride • Initiator: Light and dark cure systems; camphorquinone, two reducing agents and potassium persulphate • Others: Polycarboxylic acid, iron oxide pigments, water, titanium dioxide pigments, and stabilizer	77 wt% 58 vol%	Several in vitro studies suggest superior mechanical properties and dentin bond strength compared to conventional giomers but inferior to conventional resin composite counterparts [1–3, 13–15]

GPDMA glycerol-phosphate dimethacrylate, *HEMA* hydroxyethylmethacrylate, *Bis-GMA* bisphenol-A-glycidyl methacrylate, *UDMA* urethane dimethacrylate, *TEG-DMA* triethylenglycoldimethacrylate, *4-META* 4-methacryloxyethyl trimellitic acid

10.2 Ion Release, Bioactive, and Antibacterial Properties of Resin-Based Bulk-Fill Materials

The widespread popularity of GI-based materials is largely attributed to their fluoride ion release and uptake. GI-based materials exhibit anticariogenic properties owing to the bacteriostatic effect of fluoride ions and the increased resistance of hard tissues containing fluoride to acid dissolution [16]. Several materials have recently been developed in order to preserve the simplicity of application, ion release and cariostatic properties whilst mitigating the shortcomings associated with GI-based materials such as poor aesthetics and reduced mechanical properties. Furthermore, the adoption of the biomimetic approach in various disciplines in dentistry has fuelled the development of bioactive restoratives. The objective of such bioactive restoratives is to overcome the drawbacks associated with amalgam alternatives, namely marginal gap and microleakage.

10.2.1 Resin Composites with Alkaline Fillers

Bioactive materials can be defined as materials that can affect a biological process, namely remineralisation of dental hard tissues, as a result of the interaction with the surrounding environment. In restorative materials, the bioactive glass filler system is the reactive component and responsible for releasing, upon degradation at neutral pH, calcium, and phosphate ions leading to the formation of an apatite-like phase to fill the marginal gap [17]. Ion release is also associated with pH buffering in acidic environment especially if the bioactive filler contains an alkaline component. Activa bioactive restorative (AB; Pulpdent, USA) is a heavily marketed resin-containing, bioactive bulk-fill restorative. AB was claimed to exhibit self-adhesive properties owing to the ionic interaction between phosphate acid groups within the so-called ionic resin matrix and calcium ions within the tooth structure. Furthermore, the manufacturer asserts that the bioactive glass filler system promotes mineral apatite formation and remineralisation at the restoration-tooth interface. However, several in vitro studies have cast doubt on AB's performance. The self-adhesiveness of AB was deemed nonexistent in one study [18], others reported a significantly lower bond strength to enamel and dentin as compared to conventional resin composites and other self-adhering restoratives [13, 14, 19]. Furthermore, AB exhibited lower wear resistance when compared to conventional resin composites [2]. Clinical data regarding the performance of AB is mixed, one study demonstrated poor treatment outcomes (annual failure rate = 24.1%) and the primary cause of failure was loss of retention followed by post-operative symptoms and secondary caries [20]. In contrast, another study reported comparable, short-term clinical performance of AB and a nanohybrid resin composite [21]. Regarding the bioactivity, one study demonstrated lack of glass degradation and apatite formation with AB under different experimental conditions [22]. Another study revealed that AB underscores a conventional RMGI based bulk-fill restorative in terms of fluoride release [23]. Rigorous in vitro verification of the performance of AB is warranted in order to determine the clinical benefits and the scope of indications for such material in clinical practice.

Alkasite, a recently introduced tooth-coloured restorative material which is comprised of alkaline fillers embedded in a resin matrix. Cention N (CN; Ivoclar Vivadent, Germany) is a commercially available alkasite processed by hand mixing powder and liquid. Its application requires the use of an adhesive bond in non-retentive cavity preparations hence it is not considered a self-adhering material. The currently-available evidence suggests that using adhesive bonding with CN results in less microleakage [24] and improves bond strength to dentin acting as an intermediary reliever of polymerisation stresses [1]. The material is primarily self-cured and utilizes thiocarbamide, hydroperoxide and copper salt as chemical initiators. Light curing of CN is optional but effective to accelerate the setting of the surface layer (4 mm) of the material. The photoinitiator system is comprised of a dibenzoyel germanium derivative (Ivocerin) and an acyl phosphine oxide. Ivocerin exhibits a higher photocuring reactivity and light-absorption in the 400–450 nm wavelength range as compared to camphoroquinone [1, 25]. CN contains four different dimethacrylate based monomers and urethane dimethacrylate is the main component of the monomeric matrix. The monomer matrix comprises approximately 12–40 (wt%) of the set material. The powder contains the inorganic fillers (particle size: 0.1–35 μm, 78.4 wt%) including barium aluminium silicate glass filler, ytterbium trifluoride, an isofiller, calcium barium aluminium fluorosilicate, and calcium fluorsilicate. The last two fillers are primarily responsible for the ion release exhibited by this material. Calcium fluorsilicate, the alkaline filler comprises 24.6 (wt%) of the set material and is responsible for calcium, hydroxyl, and fluoride ion release [26]. Hydroxyl ions released from CN can play an important role in neutralizing acidic conditions generated by cariogenic flora or acidic foods and drinks. Further, hydroxyl ions may lead to higher plaque pH thus reducing the demineralisation potential of biofilm in the vicinity of the restoration [27]. CN releases calcium and fluoride ions and forms an apatite-like phase upon immersion in artificial saliva (pH = 7.0) [22]. An in vitro study revealed that CN (self-cured) has the highest fluoride ion release and alkalizing potential in acidic pH as compared to CN (light-cured) and a GI-based material [28]. Furthermore, CN was associated with higher fluoride ion release and recharge capacity when compared to other GI-based materials [29, 30]. CN was also associated with significantly smaller demineralised areas in enamel and dentin following an artificial caries challenge as compared to a conventional resin composite material [31]. Despite having a rougher surface following finishing procedure, CN exhibited lower S. mutans adhesion as compared to a smoother resin composite counterpart [32]. In the light of the presented evidence, CN meets the criteria of a bioactive material and can potentially reduce microleakage and might be of a significant clinical benefit owing to the anticariogenic potential. However, several aspects regarding the bioactivity of CN are yet to be thoroughly investigated especially the effects of using an adhesive resin with the material on the ion release and uptake potential.

CN exhibited a higher degree of conversion compared to a hybrid resin composite restorative [33]. Furthermore, it exhibited comparable dentin shear bond strength to a nano-hybrid [34] and a flowable bulk-fill [35] resin composites when all used materials bonded to dentin using etch-rinse-bond. Moreover, CN exhibited significantly higher microtensile bond strength to dentin when compared to a RMGI material [1]. CN demonstrates superior mechanical, aesthetic, and marginal sealing properties when compared to conventional GI and RMGI restoratives [33, 36]. When compared to hybrid resin composite restorative, CN demonstrated lower microleakage and inferior flexural strength [36]. The high ion release of CN may indicate increased susceptibility of the filler system to acid attack and hydrolysis which in turn, may reduce wear resistance [22]. Thus, it might be prudent to veneer CN with a conventional resin composite restorative in load bearing areas. Alternatively, additional light curing of the occlusal surface restored with CN may significantly reduce material wear as demonstrated in one in vitro study [37].

10.2.2 Resin Composites with Fluoride-Containing Filler Systems

Incorporation of fluoride containing filler systems in resin composites has long been done in order to exploit the anticariogenic potential of the former. However, a limited number of such resin composite restoratives can be used for bulk-fill application (increment thickness ≥4 mm). Tetric EvoCeram Bulk Fill (TEC; Ivoclar Vivadent, Germany) is one example on fluoride releasing bulk-fill resin composites. The proprietary filler system in TEC is largely responsible for the low polymerisation shrinkage associated with such a material. Ytterbium trifluoride is the filler component responsible for the fluoride release in TEC. Despite lower fluoride ion release compared to conventional GI materials [38], TEC exhibited significantly less demineralisation around restoration margins when compared to a non-fluoride releasing resin composite [39].

Other fluoride containing fillers may include the GI type filler (Fluoro-Alumino-Silicate) and CaF_2 nanoparticles [40]. CaF_2 nanoparticles are synthesized via spray-drying and capable of releasing high concentrations of fluoride ions [40]. Experimental resin composites containing CaF_2 exhibited high release of calcium and fluoride ions as well as potent biofilm inhibition as indicated by the low production of lactic acid, and the decreased colony forming unit [41]. The virtue of using CaF_2 nanoparticles is the fact that antibacterial properties and fluoride release occurs at low fillers concentrations (20–30% by mass). This indicates that the bioactivity of such compound can be exploited whilst allowing for incorporation of other strengthening or reinforcing fillers to be used to configure resin composites with optimum mechanical properties. Therefore, incorporating CaF_2 nanoparticles could revolutionize bulk-fill resin composites to produce highly bioactive, caries resistant and yet durable bulk-fill restoratives. Table 10.2: Summary of chemical composition and literature pertaining to some commercially available bioactive, ion-releasing bulk-fill resin-based composites.

Table 10.2 Bioactive and ion-releasing resin composites

Materials	Manufacturer	Chemical composition	Filler load	Research data
Activa bioactive	Pulpdent	• Filler: Bioactive glass, amorphous silica, sodium fluoride • Resin: Blend of diurethane and methacrylates with modified polyacrylic acid • Photoinitiator: Camphorquinone	Not specified	In vitro studies demonstrated suboptimal mechanical properties and bond strength to tooth structure [2, 13, 14, 19]. Bioactivity was deemed nonexistent by one in vitro study [22]. Clinical studies are short-term with mixed outcomes [20, 21]
Cention N	Ivoclar Vivadent	• liquid: UDMA, DCP, PEG-400 DMA hydroperoxide initiator, stabilizers and additives • Powder: Barium aluminium silicate glass, ytterbium trifluoride, isofiller, calcium barium aluminium fluorosilicate glass, calcium fluorosilicate glass calcium, thiocarbamide initiator, copper salt accelerator, and pigments • Photoinitiator: Ivocerin	Wt: Up to ≈ 78%	Strong alkalizing potential and high fluoride release [22, 27, 28]. The use of adhesive bonding with Cention N resulted in less microleakage and higher dentin bond strength [24, 34, 35]
Tetric EvoCeram bulk fill	Ivoclar Vivadent	• Resin: Bis-GMA, Bis-EMA, UDMA • Filler: Barium aluminium silicate glass, ytterbium trifluoride, mixed oxide, prepolymers, additives • Photoinitiator: Camphorquinone, acyl phosphine oxide, Ivocerin	Wt: 81% Vol: 61%	Lower demineralization around restorations compared to conventional resin composite materials [39]

UDMA urethane dimethacrylate, *DCP* tricyclodecan-dimethanol dimethacrylate PEG-400 DMA, polyethylene glycol 400 dimethacrylate, *Bis-GMA* bisphenol-A-glycidylmethacrylate, *Bis-EMA* ethyoxylated bisphenol A dimethacrylate

10.2.3 Resin Composites with Novel/Experimental Filler Systems

Amorphous calcium phosphate (ACP) nanoparticles have demonstrated promising potential for long-lasting calcium and phosphate ion release. One study reported the use of UDMA and triethylene glycol divinylbenzyl ether (TEG-DVBE), 3% dimethylaminohexadecyl methacrylate (DMAHDM), and 20% ACP nanoparticles to produce an antibacterial and bioactive low-shrinkage resin composite [42]. DMAHDM possess strong antibacterial activity, TEG-DVBE exhibits lower susceptibility to enzymatic and hydrolytic degradation, UDMA is a high molecular weight structural monomer that higher exhibits high stability toward salivary hydrolysis, greater flexibility, and cross-linking density which confer improved mechanical properties and low polymerisation shrinkage [42]. The ACP experimental resin composite achieved substantial long-term (3 months) antibacterial activity as indicated by the significant reduction of S. mutans biofilm colony-forming units and lactic acid production. Furthermore, high resistance to S. mutans biofilm acidic attack was observed with the experimental ACP resin composite as indicated by the significantly higher dentin hardness in the vicinity of dentin-composite interface as compared to a conventional resin composite restorative. The ACP experimental resin composite exhibited significantly lower polymerization shrinkage stress and similar mechanical properties as compared to a conventional resin composite restorative [42]. However, the study did not specify as to whether this experimental material can be used for bulk fill or incremental application.

Other bioactive materials have been explored as potential fillers for resin composite materials. Calcium sodium phosphosilicate (Bioglass 45S5) and Portland cement have been investigated as modifiers for commercially available bulk-fill restoratives. Bioglass 45S5 (20 wt%) did not adversely affect the degree of conversion or hardness of the investigated bulk-fill restoratives. Portland cement was, however, found to have a deleterious effect on the polymerisation of the studied materials as a result of the significant drop in materials' light transmittance [43]. Niobium-containing bioactive glasses have also promising potential in the development of remineralising resin composites as they do not seem to adversely affect the degree of monomer conversion [44]. They are also associated with high mineral deposition and pulp fibroblasts viability [44]. Such findings were obtained from an in vitro study that utilized the niobium bioactive glass as filler for an adhesive resin. Further studies are required to verify the performance of bulk-fill resin composites doped with such bioactive filler.

The significant progress in biomaterial's research in bone regeneration may inspire futuristic ideas for bioactive and biocompatible bulk-fill resin composites. Currently, the utility of polymer composites has a predominant role as scaffolds in bone tissue engineering [45]. Chitosan (CS) is a bioactive polymer that exhibits high biocompatibility and antibacterial activity. It can be produced by deacetylation of chitin; a highly abundant natural polysaccharides [45, 46]. CS can be combined with hydroxyapatite, calcium phosphate, resinous materials, or ceramic particles to form strong, and yet bioactive composites [45, 46]. The controlled biodegradability and solubility in acidic environment of CS can be pivotal to achieve cariostatic properties. CS based composites are yet to be implemented in bulk-fill dental restoratives. Despite the promising properties, the impact of biodegradability on biomechanical reliability and durability of such material warrants meticulous consideration.

Carbon nanotubes (CnTs) are allotropes of carbon with a cylindrical nanostructure and constructed with length-to-diameter ratio of up to 28,000,000:1 [45]. CnTs containing composites have attracted great attention as biocompatible coatings for load-bearing orthopaedic implants [45]. CnTs enhance strength and fracture toughness of the composite materials as they exhibit high surface area, low density and exceptionally high strength and stiffness. Besides CnTs' function as a reinforcing phase to various composites, their role as carrier for bioactive ceramic materials is of a great importance. Incorporation of CnTs based composites in bulk-fill materials may lead to the development of strong and bioactive restoratives that can be effectively used for cusp replacement direct restorations in high load bearing areas. However, application of CnTs in dental resin composites is largely challenged by the difficulty to disperse CnTs within any matrix phase besides challenging production of pure forms of CnTs [45]. Absolute gap free margins seem to be far from achievable with the currently available resin composite restorations and secondary caries remains one of the leading causes for failure [47]. This is primarily related to polymerization shrinkage and placement techniques. Hence, developing material that possess bioactive, antibacterial and low polymerisation shrinkage seems to be the way forward to reduce recurrent caries and improve a restorations' longevity. Such materials can potentially improve restorations' longevity at several levels including; smaller marginal gap, lower bacterial colonization or the marginal gap, reduced demineralisation as a result of decreasing acidogenic potential of the bacterial biofilm and buffering capacity of the bioactive fillers, decreased enzymatic degradation of resin composite components and collagen fibres of dentin, and increasing the remineralisation capacity of de novo or remnants carious/demineralised lesions. Furthermore, such bioactive bulk-fill composites may have a great potential to be used as biocompatible bone cements for artificial implants. They might be a biomechanically superior alternative to conventional poly methyl methacrylate cement with a more controlled setting reaction.

10.3 Self-Healing or Crack-Sealing Properties

Bulk fracture or chipping of resin composite restorations are among the leading reasons for restoration repair or replacement [48]. In the oral environment, polymerisation shrinkage, fluctuation of temperature, and repetitive occlusal loading especially in the stress bearing areas may lead to the accumulation of cracks within the restorations. This matter is further complicated in extensive restorations or in the presence of excessive occlusal loading as a result of parafunctional habits. Once a crack propagates to a critical size/length, fracture of the restoration becomes inevitable. Thus, it is paramount to engineer restorative materials to inhibit crack growth and propagation. One of the strategies to fulfil such objective is to integrate a self-healing or a crack-sealing mechanism within the restorative material.

10.3.1 Urea-Based Capsular Shell Systems

A widely investigated self-healing mechanism is based on releasing reactive molecules from micro- or nano-capsules in response to a mechanical stimulus [49]. Such reactive molecules can repair crack damage and recover the mechanical performance of a resin matrix polymer. A recent systematic review identified ten studies and two patents describing self-healing microcapsule-based resin composite restoratives [49]. Poly urea-formaldehyde (UF), melamine-modified UF, and polyoxymethylene urea were all reported as capsular shell material whilst poly UF being the most commonly utilized. In this group of microcapsules, the healing agents used were DCPD, TEGDMA-DHEPT, TMPET, UDMA, Bis-GMA, and MBDMA amine. One study reported using melamine-modified UF with DCPD monomer and no catalyst whilst all other studies reported the use of a catalyst system such as Grubb's catalyst or benzoyl peroxide [50]. Rupture of microcapsules as a result of crack formation releases the healing monomeric molecules which become in contact with a catalyst that is dispersed within the resin composite matrix. Consequently, a polymerisation reaction leads to the formation of a reparative polymer in the vicinity of the mechanical stimulus that eventually obturate flaws created by propagating cracks.

10.3.2 Silanized Silica Microcapsule Systems

Silanized silica microcapsules have been advocated as an alternative to urea-based counterparts. Silica microcapsules exhibit a lower tendency to rupture owing to the significantly higher shell thickness as compared to poly UF counterparts (160–230 nm vs. 4–8 μm) [49]. However, silanization of the silica microcapsule increases the bond strength to the resin matrix and facilitates microcapsule rupture upon exposure to a propagating crack as well as improves the overall mechanical properties of the self-healing resin composite [49]. Silanized silica microcapsules containing an aqueous solution of polyacrylic acid is another self-healing system that can be used in resin composites [51]. Once ruptured as a result of a propagating crack, polyacrylic acid reacts with amorphous calcium phosphate and strontium fluoroaluminosilicate (healing fillers) within the resin composite to produce reparative GI molecules with an ionic crosslinking network [51] (Fig. 10.2).

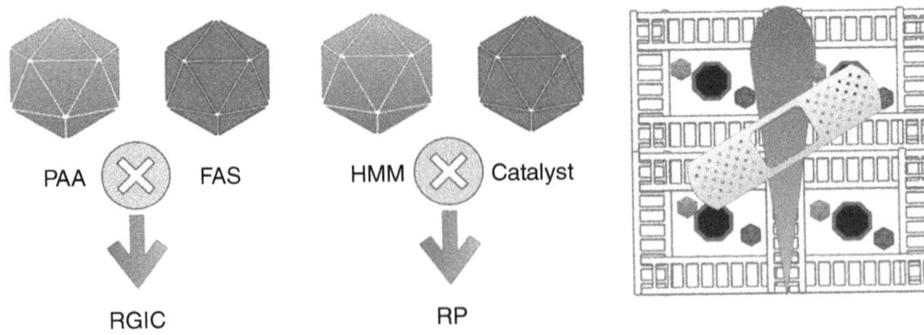

Fig. 10.2 Schematic representation of the components involved in the self-healing composite systems. *PAA* polyacrylic acid, *FAS* fluoroaluminosilicate, *RGIC* reparative glass ionomer, *HMM* hydroxy methyl methacrylate, *RP* reparative polymer

10.3.3 Potentials and Limitations of the Current Self-Healing Systems

Implementation of self-healing mechanisms is an optimum utilization of biomimetic approach to overcome a significant problem encountered with resin composite restoratives. Microcapsules loaded with various healing substances resulted in 25–80% recovery of the original fracture toughness in several experimental resin composite restoratives [49]. A significant potential is present for incorporating such technology in bulk-fill resin composites. It has been reported that microcapsules with different healing substances were able to recover the mechanical properties of various bulk, self-adhering polymeric materials with various setting mechanisms [52]. However, the exploitation of such strategy may encounter a multitude of problems related to the technicality of the production and dispersion of microcapsules within a resin composite material. Further, the instability of the catalyst compounds used in self-healing systems when subjected to high temperatures created by light curing may compromise their performance [49]. One major concern with the use of microcapsule technology is the remnant spaces created by the explosion of the microcapsules and their effects on mechanical reliability and surface roughness [49]. Concerns regarding the biocompatibility of the self-healing systems do also exist. DCPD monomer is no longer used in dental materials owing to the high cytotoxicity [53]. Local or systemic toxicity as a result of monomeric healing substance or formaldehyde elution can be of a significant concern [49]. Further research is required to ensure biosafety and efficient delivery of the healing agents in resin composite restoratives (Table 10.3).

Table 10.3 Summary of self-healing systems and their chemical composition

Capsular shell type	Chemical ingredient of healing agents	Strength recovery
PUF-microcapsules	TEGDMA-DHEPT monomers BPO catalyst	57–81%
	Bis-GMA,UDMA,TMPTMA, MBDMA BPO + PA (catalyst)	≈ 40%
	DCPD monomer Grubb's catalyst	≈ 57%
Melamine-modified UF-microcapsules	DCPD monomer	N/A
Silanized silica microcapsules	Aqueous solution of polyacrylic acid strontium fluoroaluminosilicate glass filler	≈ 25%

10.4 Aesthetic Properties

Achieving an optimum aesthetic result with direct resin composites requires meticulous placement of multiple layers with different opacities/values. In principle, this contradicts the concept of bulk filling and negates many of its advantages. Furthermore, the current bulk-fill restoratives cover basic monochromatic shades and enamel, dentine, body, translucent, and opaque shades are yet to be made available. Rather than using pigments to obtain different shades, structurally coloured resin composites utilize filler systems with refractive index similar to that for the cured resin matrix [54, 55]. This, in turn, results in sufficient light diffusivity to produce the so-called chameleon effect [55]. In one commercially available conventional resin composite (OmniChroma, Tokuyama Dental Corp., Japan), the uniformly sized supra-nano spherical zirconia and silica fillers (260 nm) reflects light in the red-to-yellow spectrum [56]. Similarly, light reflected from adjacent tooth structure is within the same spectrum. The combined light reflection from tooth structure and restoration besides the diffusion of light from the restoration into the nearby tooth structure may lead to enhanced colour matching [57]. This in turn has led to development of universal shade restoratives that could cover a wide range of classical shades.

Bulk-fill restoratives may benefit from such advances in colour chemistry where anterior teeth can be restored in bulk whilst produce an aesthetically appealing outcome. In human teeth, fluorescent emission by ambient UV light occurs primarily in dentine which is related to its organic content [58]. The bluish-white fluorescence of human teeth is the result of a broad emission band with a diffuse peak at 410–420 nm when subjected to near UV excitation [59]. Fluorescence is a key determinant of aesthetic outcome and shade match [60]. Ideal restorative materials should exhibit fluorescence similar to that of natural teeth [59, 60]. Aesthetic performance and shade match was negatively affected with restorative materials that exhibited less intense fluorescence than natural teeth [61]. Rare earth metals have been used in dental resin composites and ceramics to act as lumiphores [59]. However, they reportedly failed to yield fluorescence comparable to that of tooth structure [59]. Semiconductor nanoparticles or the so-called quantum dots may exhibit more potential in manipulation of resin composite's fluorescence. The highly luminescent, core-shell, Cadmium Selenide-Zinc Sulphide (CdSe/ZnS) composite quantum dots were able to modify the fluorescence of a conventional resin composite material to match that of natural teeth [62]. Such an approach can be of great potential to improve shade matching of bulk-fill restoratives via optimizing fluorescence intensity. However, concerns remain regarding long term performance should this approach be utilized. Several factors within the oral environment such as temperature fluctuation, enzymatic activity, moisture, and oxidation reactions may reduce quantum yield and thereby fluorescence intensity.

10.5 How to Choose from the Ever-Growing Bulk-Fill Restoratives Available to Practitioners

Clinicians have the duty to select the restorative material that meets the functional and aesthetic demands of the patient at the least biological cost and which provides the best available favourable prognosis. The vast and progressively increasing variety of dental materials in the market alongside the increased marketing activities has rendered material selection a difficult task for clinicians. Clinicians should use/update their working knowledge to scrutinize various aspects related to the properties and performance of each material. Being aware of the specifications, advantages, disadvantages, and grades of a particular dental material as well as the clinical demands of the patient is key for optimum material selection.

"The field of dental materials has grown significantly, but the time available for teaching and studying this subject has not", a statement made in one of the most famous dental materials textbooks more than a decade ago [63]. As of yet, no notable changes to the undergraduate dental curricula could be observed to accommodate the growth of this field. Thus, at the end of this book, we propose a succinct and structured strategy to help the clinicians make a balanced and evidence-based decision to select a particular restorative material.

10.5.1 Choosing Materials in the Same Category

It is always useful to compare a new material to reference counterparts or previous generations of the same material with long-term and documented optimum clinical performance. Independent and long-term clinical studies with a low risk of bias provide optimum evidence and guidance for clinicians in this context. However, with emerging, new materials such studies are scarce. Thus, it is prudent to resort to independent in vitro studies and short-term clinical trials. The findings of such studies should be scrutinized and compared to reference materials in order to make an informed decision on how well this material may perform in a clinical environment.

10.5.2 Using Marketing Data

There are several examples where extensively marketed dental materials failed to convey any advantage when rigorously tested in clinical trials. It is widely accepted that manufacturer-funded studies will very likely report less complication rates and more positive research findings. Of course, such findings can be trusted once confirmed by studies conducted by independent researchers and published in journals with a strict policy to deal with conflict of interest among researchers. Findings from studies comparing materials from the same category manufactured by different competitors can also be utilized effectively to help with material selection.

10.5.3 Moving Beyond *P*-Values

Leaving aside the controversy among statisticians regarding the validity of the statistical significance as a tool, clinicians should critically appraise research findings and their validity/relevance to clinical practice. In this context, clinicians should understand that materials with significantly superior performance over a competitor counterpart or previous generation may only provide an extra 0.2 mm of clinical attachment gain, 4% reduction in polymerisation shrinkage, or 15 s shorter procedure time, which are all barely measurable and of no clinical significance.

It is also paramount that clinicians assess whether the used methodology adequately answers the research question. In this context, clinicians differentiate between success and survival reported in clinical studies and the implications of the difference between the two outcomes on clinical decision making. In the case of in vitro studies, the burden is larger as deeper knowledge is required to extrapolate clinically relevant data. For instance, cyclic fatigue studies of restored natural teeth are more relevant to the clinical situation compared to static experimental designs utilizing disc- or beam-shaped specimens.

10.5.4 Operator's Clinical Experience and Expertise

The three pillars that comprise evidence-based dentistry are patient's needs, scientific evidence, and clinician's expertise. Whilst clinicians must endeavour to choose materials based on sound research data, they also must ensure that they master the handling of such material. Hands-on training are key to optimize clinical techniques utilizing new dental materials prior to using them for patients.

10.6 Summary

This chapter has explored the progress already achieved with bulk-fill resin composite materials but also potential improvements to this group of materials, that might lead to improved clinical outcomes have been explored in depth. The following conclusions can be drawn:

1. Self-adhering bulk materials would be a significant asset in clinical practice; however, significant research is needed to further develop these materials.
2. Bioactive or bio reactive, ion release, and antimicrobial properties are desirable characteristics for all materials but in this context for bulk-fill resin composite materials. There is much to do, however, to develop these technologies not least to demonstrate the clinical benefit.
3. Whilst self-healing and crack sealing properties are valid areas for further research there are concerns about the biosafety and the efficient delivery of these materials and again the clinical benefits need to be demonstrated in suitably designed and powered clinical trials.

4. Traditionally bulk-fill materials have performed poorly with respect to achieving a good aesthetic outcome. There are interesting, proposed developments to improve the aesthetics of this group of materials but further development and clinical evaluation is required.

References

1. Yao C, et al. Structural/chemical characterization and bond strength of a new self-adhesive bulk-fill restorative. J Adhes Dent. 2020;22(1):85–97.
2. Frankenberger R, et al. Amalgam alternatives critically evaluated: effect of long-term thermomechanical loading on marginal quality, wear, and fracture behavior. J Adhes Dent. 2020;22(1):107–16.
3. Latta MA, et al. In vitro wear resistance of self-adhesive restorative materials. J Adhes Dent. 2020;22(1):59–64.
4. Cho E, Kopel H, White SN. Moisture susceptibility of resin-modified glass-ionomer materials. Quintessence Int. 1995;26(5):351–8.
5. Bonsor SJ. Resin-based composite materials: a science update. Dent Update. 2019;46(4):304–12.
6. Rangappa A, et al. Comparative evaluation of bond strength of self-adhering flowable composites to the dentin prepared with different burs: an in vitro study. J Conserv Dent. 2018;21(6):618–21.
7. Mine A, et al. Limited interaction of a self-adhesive flowable composite with dentin/enamel characterized by TEM. Dent Mater. 2017;33(2):209–17.
8. Maj A, et al. A comparative clinical study of the self-adhering flowable composite resin vertise flow and the traditional flowable composite resin premise flowable. Coatings. 2020;10(8):800.
9. Peterson J, et al. Bonding performance of self-adhesive flowable composites to enamel, dentin and a nano-hybrid composite. Odontology. 2018;106(2):171–80.
10. Poitevin A, et al. Bonding effectiveness of self-adhesive composites to dentin and enamel. Dent Mater. 2013;29(2):221–30.
11. Celik EU, Aka B, Yilmaz F. Six-month clinical evaluation of a self-adhesive flowable composite in noncarious cervical lesions. J Adhes Dent. 2015;17(4):361–8.
12. Hanabusa M, et al. TEM interfacial characterization of an experimental self-adhesive filling material bonded to enamel/dentin. Dent Mater. 2011;27(8):818–24.
13. Latta MA, et al. Enamel and dentin bond durability of self-adhesive restorative materials. J Adhes Dent. 2020;22(1):99–105.
14. Latta MA, Radniecki SM. Bond strength of self-adhesive restorative materials affected by smear layer thickness but not dentin desiccation. J Adhes Dent. 2020;22(1):79–84.
15. Lohbauer U, Belli R. The mechanical performance of a novel self-adhesive restorative material. J Adhes Dent. 2020;22(1):47–58.
16. Larsen M, Bruun C. Caries chemistry and fluoride-mechanisms of action. In: Textbook of clinical cariology. Copenhagen, Denmark: Munksgaard; 1994. p. 231–54.
17. Jun S-K, Lee J-H, Lee H-H. The biomineralization of a bioactive glass-incorporated light-curable pulp capping material using human dental pulp stem cells. Biomed Res Int. 2017;2017:2495282.
18. Benetti AR, et al. Adhesion and marginal adaptation of a claimed bioactive, restorative material. Biomater Investig Dent. 2019;6(1):90–8.
19. Alkhudhairy FI, Z.H. Ahmad comparison of shear bond strength and microleakage of various bulk-fill bioactive dentin substitutes: an in vitro study. J Contemp Dent Pract. 2016;17:997–1002.
20. van Dijken JW, Pallesen U, Benetti A. A randomized controlled evaluation of posterior resin restorations of an altered resin modified glass-ionomer cement with claimed bioactivity. Dent Mater. 2019;35(2):335–43.

21. Bhadra D, et al. A 1-year comparative evaluation of clinical performance of nanohybrid composite with Activa™ bioactive composite in class II carious lesion: a randomized control study. J Conserv Dent. 2019;22(1):92–6.
22. Tiskaya M, et al. Characterization of the bioactivity of two commercial composites. Dent Mater. 2019;35(12):1757–68.
23. Garoushi S, Vallittu PK, Lassila L. Characterization of fluoride releasing restorative dental materials. Dent Mater J. 2018;37(2):293–300. advpub
24. Mazumdar P, Das A, Das U. Comparative evaluation of microleakage of three different direct restorative materials (silver amalgam, glass ionomer cement, Cention N), in class II restorations using stereomicroscope: an in vitro study. Indian J Dent Res. 2019;30(2):277–81.
25. Moszner N, et al. Benzoyl germanium derivatives as novel visible light photo initiators for dental materials. Dent Mater. 2008;24(7):901–7.
26. Todd J. Scientific documentation: Cention N. Schaan, Liechtenstein: Ivoclar-Vivadent Press; 2016. p. 1–58.
27. Persson A, Lingstrom P, van Dijken JW. Effect of a hydroxyl ion-releasing composite resin on plaque acidogenicity. Caries Res. 2005;39(3):201–6.
28. Gupta N, et al. Comparison of fluoride ion release and alkalizing potential of a new bulk-fill alkasite. J Conserv Dent. 2019;22(3):296–9.
29. Rai S, Kumari RA, Meena N. Comparative assessment of fluoride release and recharge through newer fluoride releasing posterior restorative materials: an in vitro study. J Conserv Dent. 2019;22(6):544.
30. Ruengrungsom C, et al. Evaluation of F, Ca, and P release and microhardness of eleven ion-leaching restorative materials and the recharge efficacy using a new Ca/P containing fluoride varnish. J Dent. 2020;102:103474.
31. Donly KJ, Liu JA. Dentin and enamel demineralization inhibition at restoration margins of vitremer, Z 100 and Cention N. Am J Dent. 2018;31(3):166–8.
32. Park C, et al. Surface roughness and microbial adhesion after finishing of Alkasite restorative material. J Korean Acad Pediatr Dent. 2020;47(2):188–95.
33. Panpisut P, Toneluck A. Monomer conversion, dimensional stability, biaxial flexural strength, and fluoride release of resin-based restorative material containing alkaline fillers. Dent Mater J. 2020;39(4):608–15. advpub
34. Naz F, et al. Comparative evaluation of mechanical and physical properties of a new bulk-fill alkasite with conventional restorative materials. Saudi Dent J. 2020;33(7):666–73.
35. Awad MM, et al. Evaluation of the bond strength and cytotoxicity of alkasite restorative material. Appl Sci. 2020;10(18):6175.
36. Sujith R, et al. Comparative evaluation of mechanical and microleakage properties of Cention-N, composite, and glass ionomer cement restorative materials. J Contemp Dent Pract. 2020;21(6):691–5.
37. Roulet J-F, et al. In vitro wear of dual-cured bulkfill composites and flowable bulkfill composites. J Esthet Restor Dent. 2020;32(5):512–20.
38. Naoum S, et al. Fluoride release, recharge and mechanical property stability of various fluoride-containing resin composites. Oper Dent. 2011;36(4):422–32.
39. Leon-Pineda C, Donly K. Inhibition of demineralization at restoration margins of Z100 and tetric EvoCeram bulk fill in dentin and enamel. Bioengineering. 2019;6(2):36.
40. Xu H, et al. Novel CaF2 nanocomposite with high strength and fluoride ion release. J Dent Res. 2010;89(7):739–45.
41. Mitwalli H, et al. Novel CaF2 nanocomposites with antibacterial function and fluoride and calcium ion release to inhibit oral biofilm and protect teeth. J Funct Biomater. 2020;11(3):56.
42. Bhadila G, et al. Bioactive low-shrinkage-stress nanocomposite suppresses S. mutans biofilm and preserves tooth dentin hardness. Acta Biomater. 2020;114:146–57.
43. Dieckmann P, et al. Light transmittance and polymerization of bulk-fill composite materials doped with bioactive micro-fillers. Materials (Basel). 2019;12(24):4087.
44. Balbinot GDS, et al. Niobium containing bioactive glasses as remineralizing filler for adhesive resins. Dent Mater. 2020;36(2):221–8.

45. Venkatesan J, Kim SK. Chitosan composites for bone tissue engineering—an overview. Mar Drugs. 2010;8(8):2252–66.
46. Muxika A, et al. Chitosan as a bioactive polymer: processing, properties and applications. Int J Biol Macromol. 2017;105(Pt 2):1358–68.
47. Demarco FF, et al. Longevity of posterior composite restorations: not only a matter of materials. Dent Mater. 2012;28(1):87–101.
48. Opdam NJM, et al. A retrospective clinical study on longevity of posterior composite and amalgam restorations. Dent Mater. 2007;23(1):2–8.
49. Althaqafi KA, Satterthwaite J, Silikas N. A review and current state of autonomic self-healing microcapsules-based dental resin composites. Dent Mater. 2020;36(3):329–42.
50. Then S, Neon GS, Abu Kasim NH. Performance of melamine modified urea–formaldehyde microcapsules in a dental host material. J Appl Polym Sci. 2011;122(4):2557–62.
51. Huyang G, Debertin AE, Sun J. Design and development of self-healing dental composites. Mater Des. 2016;94:295–302.
52. Blaiszik BJ, et al. Microcapsules filled with reactive solutions for self-healing materials. Polymer. 2009;50(4):990–7.
53. Bevan C, et al. Subchronic toxicity study of dicyclopentadiene vapor in rats. Toxicol Ind Health. 1992;8(6):353–67.
54. Ota M, et al. Influence of refractive index on optical parameters of experimental resin composites. Acta Odontol Scand. 2012;70(5):362–7.
55. Oivanen M, et al. The effect of refractive index of fillers and polymer matrix on translucency and color matching of dental resin composite. Biomater Investig Dent. 2021;8(1):48–53.
56. Tokuyama. Omnichroma: technical report; 2021. p. 4–9.
57. Tsubone M, et al. Color shifting at the border of resin composite restorations in human tooth cavity. Dent Mater. 2012;28(8):811–7.
58. Lee YK. Fluorescence properties of human teeth and dental calculus for clinical applications. J Biomed Opt. 2015;20(4):040901.
59. Monsénégo G, Burdairon G, Clerjaud B. Fluorescence of dental porcelain. J Prosthet Dent. 1993;69(1):106–13.
60. Volpato CAM, Pereira MRC, Silva FS. Fluorescence of natural teeth and restorative materials, methods for analysis and quantification: a literature review. J Esthet Restor Dent. 2018;30(5):397–407.
61. Lee YK, Lu H, Powers JM. Influence of fluorescent and opalescent properties of resin composites on the masking effect. J Biomed Mater Res B Appl Biomater. 2006;76(1):26–32.
62. Alves LP, et al. Core-shell quantum dots tailor the fluorescence of dental resin composites. J Dent. 2010;38(2):149–52.
63. O'Brien WJ. Dental materials and their selection. Batavia, IL: Quintessence; 2008.

GPSR Compliance
The European Union's (EU) General Product Safety Regulation (GPSR) is a set of rules that requires consumer products to be safe and our obligations to ensure this.

If you have any concerns about our products, you can contact us on

ProductSafety@springernature.com

In case Publisher is established outside the EU, the EU authorized representative is:

Springer Nature Customer Service Center GmbH
Europaplatz 3
69115 Heidelberg, Germany

www.ingramcontent.com/pod-product-compliance
Ingram Content Group UK Ltd.
Pitfield, Milton Keynes, MK11 3LW, UK
UKHW020239061126
16351UKWH00016B/52
* 9 7 8 3 0 3 1 1 6 3 8 9 0 *